1-22-74

Law and Ethics of
A.I.D. and Embryo Transfer

The Ciba Foundation for the promotion of international cooperation in medical and chemical research is a scientific and educational charity established by CIBA Limited – now CIBA-GEIGY Limited – of Basle. The Foundation operates independently in London under English trust law.

Ciba Foundation Symposia are published in collaboration with Associated Scientific Publishers (Elsevier Scientific Publishing Company, Excerpta Medica, North-Holland Publishing Company) in Amsterdam.

Associated Scientific Publishers, P.O. Box 211, Amsterdam

Law and Ethics of A.I.D. and Embryo Transfer

Ciba Foundation Symposium 17 (new series)

1973

Elsevier · Excerpta Medica · North-Holland
Associated Scientific Publishers · Amsterdam · London · New York

ISBN Excerpta Medica 90 219 4018 3
ISBN American Elsevier 0-444-15014-5

Library of Congress Catalog Card Number 73-80904

Published in 1973 by Associated Scientific Publishers, P.O. Box 211, Amsterdam, and 52 Vanderbilt Avenue, New York, N.Y. 10017.
Suggested series entry for library catalogues: Ciba Foundation Symposia.

Ciba Foundation Symposium 17 (new series)

Printed in The Netherlands by Mouton & Co., The Hague

Contents

Participants

Symposium on Legal and Other Aspects of Artificial Insemination by Donor (A.I.D.) and Embryo Transfer held at the Ciba Foundation, London, 1st December 1972

I. ANDREJEW   Professor of Criminal Law, Warsaw University, Ul. Śniadeckich 12 m 70, Warsaw 10, Poland

D. C. A. BEVIS   Consultant Obstetrician and Gynaecologist, Jessop Hospital for Women, Sheffield S3 7RE

G. R. DUNSTAN   Professor of Moral and Social Theology, King's College, The Strand, London WC2R 2LS

J. H. EDWARDS   Professor of Human Genetics, Infant Development Unit, Birmingham Maternity Hospital, Birmingham B15 2TG

R. G. EDWARDS   Lecturer, Physiological Laboratory, Cambridge CB2 3EG

C. FEILDING   Emeritus Professor of Moral Theology, Trinity College, Hoskin Avenue, Toronto 181, Ontario, Canada

C. FRIED   Professor of Law, Harvard University, Cambridge, Massachussetts 02138 USA

P. J. GRAHAM   Consultant in Psychological Medicine, The Hospital for Sick Children, Great Ormond Street, London WC1N 3JH

HILDE T. HIMMELWEIT   Professor of Psychology, The London School of Economics and Political Science, Houghton Street, London WC2A 2AE

SUSANNA ISAACS   Physician in charge, Department of Child Psychiatry, St Mary's Hospital, Praed Street, Paddington, London W2 1NY

LORD KILBRANDON   Lord of Appeal in Ordinary, 2 Raymond Buildings, Gray's Inn, London WC1

ANNE MCLAREN   Hon. Lecturer, Department of Genetics, Institute of Animal
Genetics, University of Edinburgh, West Mains Road, Edinburgh
EH9 3JN

BRIDGETT A. MASON   Clinical Assistant, Infertility Unit, Royal Free Hospital,
Gray's Inn Road, London WC1X 8LF

SIR ALAN PARKES   Professor emeritus of Reproductive Physiology, Cambridge

M. F. PERUTZ   Chairman, MRC Laboratory of Molecular Biology,
University Postgraduate Medical School, Hills Road, Cambridge CB2 2QH

E. E. PHILIPP   Consultant Obstetrician and Gynaecologist, Royal Northern
Hospital, Holloway Road, London N7

M. PIATTELLI-PALMARINI   Assistant Director, Centre International d'Etudes
Bioanthropologiques et d'Anthropologie Fondamentale, Fondation
Royaumont, 23bis, rue de l'Assomption, Paris 16e, France

MARIEL REVILLARD   Centre de Recherches, d'Information et de
Documentation Notariales, CRIDON, 58 bvd des Belges, F-69 Lyon 6e,
France

SIR JOHN STALLWORTHY   Nuffield Professor of Obstetrics and Gynaecology,
John Radcliffe Hospital, Headington, Oxford OX3 9DU

P. C. STEPTOE   Senior Consultant Obstetrician and Gynaecologist,
Oldham & District General Hospital, Rochdale Road, Oldham,
Lancashire

OLIVE M. STONE   Reader in Law, The London School of Economics and
Political Science, Houghton Street, London WC2A 2AE

B. A. O. WILLIAMS   Professor of Philosophy, King's College, Cambridge
CB2 1ST

Editors: G. E. W. WOLSTENHOLME and DAVID W. FITZSIMONS

Chairman's introduction

LORD KILBRANDON

The subject matter of this conference first occurred to me during a conference run by the Institute of Society Ethics and The Life Sciences at the Fogarty International Centre in October 1971. Artificial insemination by donor (A.I.D.) was by no means the main topic of that conference but the legal status of A.I.D. is to some extent obscure and it was thought that it would be useful to clarify the position and to discuss the subject fully, not only in a legal context. Thus at this symposium we have not only lawyers but also scientists and philosophers.

Speaking as a lawyer, I must confess that compared with the medical or ethical sciences, the law is a blunt instrument, and I am not sure how helpful the legal contribution is going to be. Law, in connection with some activity of this kind, is rather inclined to resolve itself into the question 'is it *illegal?*' rather than 'is it legal?'. Fundamentally, everything is legal unless it is illegal. To that extent, the lawyer must take a rather detached view of this kind of discussion.

No doubt we shall be discussing two legal aspects, criminal and civil. Should the State prevent certain actions by criminal sanctions? Are certain actions undesirable from the point of view of the personal rights of other citizens, and therefore unlawful? This is the civil aspect. If the legal attitude appears to be generally related to prohibition, I am afraid this is inevitable if the law is to be concerned only with restraining by regulation what would otherwise have been done without reference to the law. I do not want to be discouraging in the least, because I shall be listening very carefully and hopefully. Unfortunately I am, as it were, the potential representative of the prohibitive aspect. But as a legal philosopher my personal attitude is—why not? When talking about the legal aspect of A.I.D., the legal philosopher, as contrasted with the legislator, immediately asks what is against it? To that limited extent, perhaps the legal attitude may be said to be helpful.

Biological aspects of A.I.D.

ANNE McLAREN*

The problems that artificial insemination by donor (A.I.D.) raises are not, in the main, biological. My task is therefore merely to put before you as briefly as possible the present realities of A.I.D., and to describe its direct biological consequences and certain more indirect consequences, in order to try and remove any misapprehensions at the scientific level.

PRESENT REALITIES

Artificial insemination, first used in women by John Hunter at the end of the eighteenth century, is a simple procedure from the medical point of view (see ref. 10). Semen is obtained by masturbation and is deposited by means of a syringe in or near the cervix of the woman's uterus. Since the lifespan of spermatozoa in the female reproductive tract is short, the timing of insemination is critical. The time of maximal fertility coincides with ovulation, when the egg is shed, but unfortunately at present no certain method exists for determining the time of ovulation in our own species. The date of the last menstrual period gives only a rough guide; a rise in body temperature is a useful but by no means infallible indication that the egg has been shed; examination of cells from the vagina gives additional information; changes in hormone concentrations in the blood and urine could potentially provide a more precise answer.

Because of the problem of timing, insemination on several successive days in the month increases the chances of pregnancy, but this may not always be practicable. A success rate of 70–75% pregnancies within three to four months of the start of treatment has been achieved in several centres, each series including over 200 pregnancies (for a review see ref. 2).

*I thank the Ford Foundation for financial support and also Dr Margaret Jackson for allowing me to quote her unpublished data.

Biologically, it is largely irrelevant whether the semen is provided by the husband (A.I.H.) or by a donor (A.I.D.). Here we shall be concerned mainly with A.I.D., on account of the psychological, ethical and legal problems that it poses. A.I.D. is only used when the husband is wholly infertile owing to the virtual absence of live spermatozoa from the semen, or more rarely in cases of severe rhesus incompatibility or where the husband is known to suffer from or carry some serious hereditary disease, such as Huntington's chorea or haemophilia.

In the United Kingdom and the United States, some 12% of couples have an infertility problem, and in 10–15% of these the man is wholly responsible. The potential application of A.I.D. is therefore large. The number of inseminations performed is unknown: no A.I.D. register exists in any country, mainly because of the uncertain legal status of the procedure. Schellen[12] estimated in 1957 that in the U.S. 100 000 babies had already been born as a result of artificial insemination (mainly A.I.D.), while Behrman[2] quoted a figure of 5000–10 000 births after A.I.D. for 1966 alone. In one Tokyo clinic, several hundred inseminations are performed annually.[5] In the U.K., perhaps 30 or 40 doctors practise A.I.D., some of them only operating on a few women a year, sometimes on the National Health Service. Dr Margaret Jackson, one of the pioneers of A.I.D. in England, treated 500 women between 1941 and the end of 1971. At present, A.I.D. is only considered for those couples who themselves request it: if the procedure were more widely known and information on it freely provided in infertility clinics, the number of requests would presumably increase.

BIOLOGICAL CONSEQUENCES

The major biological anxiety over any form of intervention with the reproductive process is of course that the children born might be in some way defective. With artificial insemination this fear seems groundless. One solid reassurance is provided by the massive scale on which artificial insemination is now used in cattle breeding. As early as 1780, Spallanzani had successfully inseminated a bitch, but it was not until the Second World War that artificial insemination was introduced into British agriculture, thanks largely to the energy and enthusiasm of John Hammond.[4] At the end of the 1950s, the Milk Marketing Board gave a banquet to celebrate the artificial insemination of the ten-millionth cow in the U.K. In 1969–1970, 2 645 000 cows were artificially inseminated in this country, representing about 60% of all cattle matings.[8] The practice of artificial insemination would never have spread so rapidly if there had been any indication that it might result in malformation or deterioration of the stock.

Human babies born after artificial insemination show no increase in neonatal mortality or in congenital defect. Few follow-up studies of later development have been done, perhaps because doctors do not want to risk revealing that the children have not been conceived normally. However, Iizuka et al.[5] investigated 54 A.I.D. children and found that their physical and mental development was in no way inferior to a similar control series: indeed in I.Q., which is strongly affected by the family environment, they significantly exceeded the control level.

A priori one would expect A.I.D. babies to show less mortality and fewer congenital defects than normal. Some chromosomal abnormalities are thought to arise from the fertilization of stale eggs, that is eggs which have been ovulated a day or two before insemination.[1] Intercourse in our species may take place throughout the cycle, with only a slight tendency for the incidence to increase during the fertile period; with artificial insemination, on the other hand, considerable efforts are made to synchronize insemination and ovulation, so the risk of fertilization of stale eggs is correspondingly diminished.

DEEP-FREEZE STORAGE

Recently the use of frozen semen for A.I.D. has become increasingly common. The methods used follow those pioneered by Parkes and his collaborators, namely the addition of glycerol, slow cooling, rapid freezing and storage below $-79\,°C$. Bull semen deep-frozen in this way gives a conception rate within 1–2% of that achieved with fresh semen and can be preserved for at least ten years, perhaps indefinitely. The advantages for cattle breeding are many: it facilitates semen transport over long distances, reduces the administrative problems of insemination, greatly increases the number of cows that can be inseminated from a single bull, and makes possible the testing of the progeny of the bulls before their semen is used on a large scale.

Human semen can also be stored at low temperatures, but its fertilizing capacity appears to decline faster than that of cattle semen. Tests so far[2] indicate that pregnancy rate is no more than 50% after storage for several months, compared with the 70–75% reported for fresh semen. Margaret Jackson has obtained 15 live births from A.I.D. using deep-frozen semen, with an average of 19 inseminations per birth, compared with seven inseminations per birth for fresh semen. Probably the lifespan of human spermatozoa in the female reproductive tract is reduced by storage in the cold. Development after fertilization seems to be entirely normal. Efforts to find optimum conditions for storage of human semen are being made[11] by examining the effect of different protective agents over different temperature ranges, and different rates of freezing and thawing. A mixture of glycerol, egg yolk and antibiotics seems to provide a suitable protective medium, and best results are obtained by slow cooling (1 °C/ min) from room temperature to 0 °C, faster cooling (5–7 °C/min) from 0 to −30 °C (in order to pass through the range of heat of fusion within three minutes) and still faster cooling below −30 °C. The rate of thawing appears to be less critical. Storage at −79 °C (solid carbon dioxide) is probably less satisfactory than storage at −196.5 °C (liquid nitrogen). Experiments on freeze-drying of semen are also in progress.

Long-term storage of semen has some of the same advantages for human insemination as it has for cattle breeding, namely ease of transport and administrative convenience. In 1971 a number of Californian women were inseminated with deep-frozen semen from their husbands in Vietnam. The factor of administrative convenience is an important one, particularly in view of the need to carry out inseminations during the short fertile period. Many couples want a second or even third A.I.D. child, and often prefer to use the same donor: this may be hard to arrange unless several semen samples have been deep-frozen initially. In the United States, banks for frozen semen, often run commercially, are now common. Many of their clients are men about to undergo a vasectomy, for whom a stored semen sample provides insurance against any future change of mind or circumstance. Such banks are also widely used for A.I.D., since they offer semen from a range of donors of different blood groups and physical characteristics, allowing the doctor considerable scope in 'matching' the donor to the husband. Sperm banks have found little support in England, where doctors using A.I.D. prefer to have personal knowledge of the donors.

POSSIBLE CAUSES FOR CONCERN

The problem of donor selection is an important one, which has given rise to some anxiety on various biological grounds. Fears have been expressed that willingness to become a donor might indicate some undesirable personality trait which would then be handed on to a disproportionate number of progeny. This seems an unreal cause for anxiety: leaving aside the nature of such traits and their heritability, most donors are in fact either impecunious medical students who receive a financial inducement, or the husbands of patients at a fertility clinic, who agree to act as donors out of gratitude.

Another problem is that the doctor exercises a degree of positive eugenic selection, since he only uses donors who are physically and mentally sound, with a good medical record and semen of high quality, and may introduce his own value judgements as to which personality types (for example) would make the best fathers. However, the effect of this selection would be trivial over the whole population, unless the numbers of A.I.D. progeny from an individual donor were to become very large. Some doctors try to match the donor to the husband as closely as possible; others always inseminate with a mixture of semen from different donors, so that the actual father of any given baby is unknown.

Another issue on which concern has been expressed is the possibility that A.I.D. children conceived from the same donor, and who were therefore half-brothers and half-sisters, might unwittingly marry and have children. The progeny of first-cousin marriages show a higher-than-normal mortality and malformation rate; half-brothers and half-sisters are more closely related genetically than are first cousins, so their children would be at a still greater disadvantage. However, a certain number of half-sibling marriages must take place unwittingly anyway, as a consequence of extra-marital conceptions, and the increase in their number due to A.I.D. would be expected to be very small, provided that the number of babies fathered by a single donor remained small. It has been calculated that one donor could produce enough semen for 20 000 children per year, but in practice the highest recorded number of live births from one donor is 17; most doctors set a limit at four or five. Glass[3] has estimated that, if 2000 live children a year were to be born in Great Britain as a result of the successful use of A.I.D., and if each donor were responsible for five children, an unwitting incestuous marriage is unlikely to take place more than once in 50–100 years.

If the number of children from each donor is strictly limited, not only are the risks of incestuous marriage minimized, but also any demographically undesirable effects of donor selection are avoided. A further advantage is that there will be less risk of disproportionate spread of any harmful recessive genes that the donor is carrying. In cattle breeding, where raising a large number of progeny from genetically superior bulls is one of the chief aims of artificial insemination, the hazard of wide dissemination of harmful recessive genes is very real, and carriers have to be identified through matings with their oldest daughters.

Will A.I.D. ever be used in the interests of positive eugenics, for the genetic improvement of mankind or to further some less reputable social or political aim? It is difficult to predict what will happen hundreds of years in the future, but for the next generation or two such an applications seems to me exceedingly unlikely. As I have pointed out elsewhere,[6] the principles of selective breeding have been known for centuries, but no serious attempt has ever been made to apply them to our own species. It is not easy to see why artificial insemination should be used in this way unless the structure of society changes drastically. Muller[9] argued strongly that some effort should be made to improve the quality of the human race by the use of A.I.D., but he has few supporters. Medawar[7] concluded on genetic grounds that the goal of positive eugenics could never be achieved, since 'the human genetic system does not lend itself to improvement by selective inbreeding'. We are genetically very diverse and our well-being depends on this diversity. Maynard Smith,[13] taking I.Q. score as an example, emphasized the extreme slowness of any advance under selection that could be achieved through the use of artificial insemination in women. The improvement that could be brought about by medical and educational and cultural measures would far outweigh the effects of many centuries of intense eugenic effort.

CONCLUSION

The biological problems posed by the practice of A.I.D. are not likely to be grave. Most couples want children, and will continue to do so in the foreseeable future. The increase in the incidence of contraception and abortion and the new attitudes of women in society mean that fewer and fewer babies will be available for adoption. A.I.D. therefore fills a real need, and is likely to be used more widely in the future than it is at present.

References

[1] AUSTIN, C. R. (1969) Variations and anomalies in fertilization, in *Fertilization: comparative morphology, biochemistry and immunology* (Metz, C. B. & Monroy, A., eds.), vol. 2, Academic Press, New York

[2] BEHRMAN, S. J. (1968) Techniques of artificial insemination, in *Progress in Infertility* (Behrman, S. J. & Kistner, R. W., eds.), Churchill, London

[3] GLASS, D. V. (1960) Quoted in *Report of the Departmental Committee on Human Artificial Insemination*, H.M. Stationery Office

[4] HAMMOND, J. (1962) An interview. *Journal of Reproduction and Fertility* 3, 2–13

[5] IIZUKA, R., SAWADA, Y., NISHINA, N. & OHI, M. (1968) The physical and mental development of children born following artificial insemination. *International Journal of Fertility* 13, 24–32

[6] McLAREN, A. (1971) The future of the family, in *The Future of Man (Institute of Biology Symposium no. 20)* (Ebling, F. J. & Heath, G. W., eds.), pp. 65–75, Academic Press, London & New York

[7] MEDAWAR, P. B. (1969) The genetic improvement of man. *Australasian Annals of Medicine* 4, 317–320

[8] MILK MARKETING BOARD (1969–1970) *Report of the Breeding and Production Organization*, No. 20

[9] MULLER, H. J. (1963) Genetical progress by voluntarily conducted germinal choice in *Man and his Future (Ciba Foundation Symposium)* (Wolstenholme, G., ed.), Churchill, London

[10] REPRODUCTION RESEARCH INFORMATION SERVICE (1972) Artificial insemination and freeze-preservation of human semen. *Bibliography of Reproduction* 19, 1–8, 141–146

[11] SAWADA, Y. & ACKERMAN, D. R. (1968) Use of frozen human semen in *Progress in Infertility* (Behrman, S. J. & Kistner, R. W., eds.), Churchill, London
[12] SCHELLEN, A. M. C. M. (1957) *Artificial Insemination in the Human*, Elsevier, Amsterdam
[13] SMITH, J. M. (1965) Eugenics and Utopia. *Daedalus* **94**, 487–505

Biological aspects of embryo transfer

R. G. EDWARDS and P. C. STEPTOE

Recent advances in the control of early development in mammals and man mean that it may soon be possible for human eggs to be fertilized outside the body, grown for a few days in culture and then replaced in the mother's uterus. The clinical advantages of this procedure would be immediate, for many infertile men and women, especially those with oligospermia or occluded oviducts, can be offered no therapy for their condition at present and must remain irreversibly sterile. Other advantages may include a deeper understanding of human genetic disorders and the development of new methods of contraception. Here we shall summarize present knowledge about embryo transfer in mammals[2, 8, 11] and about the fertilization and cleavage *in vitro* of human eggs.

Before we consider the biological aspects of embryo transfer, a few words are needed about the wider implications of the method. Unlike artificial insemination by donor, the legal and other problems are not immediate, for no human pregnancies or offspring after embryo transfer have yet been reported. Also the scientific and technical developments needed to establish the two methods obviously differ, as A.I.D. makes virtually no demands on scientific know-how; the same results could be achieved by adultery. But embryo transfer depends on close collaboration between doctor and scientist, and on the development of suitable methods for obtaining, growing and transferring the embryos. Another important difference is that embryo transfer will be used almost exclusively for many years to come to alleviate infertility within a marriage, by giving husbands and wives a chance to have their own children. Relatively few women need an oocyte or an embryo from a donor to alleviate their infertility; such treatment will be limited to only a small number of patients.

EMBRYO TRANSFER IN ANIMALS

The first embryo transfer was performed between rabbits as long ago as 1890,[21] and by now embryos in all stages of their preimplantation development have been transferred after culture for various periods of time. Eggs or embryos in various early stages of their development have been successfully transferred in seven or more mammalian species. Although both one-celled eggs, whether fertilized or unfertilized, and two-celled eggs are usually placed in the oviduct, those in later stages are returned to the uterus. The stage at which the embryo enters the uterus naturally varies from species to species; it occurs as early as the four-cell stage in pigs and much later in other species. Human embryos probably enter the uterus between the 8-cell and the 16-cell stage.

The stage of development of the embryo and the endocrine status of the recipient must be matched during embryo transfers. In mice and rabbits, the incidence of successful transfers is greatly reduced if the embryo is one day 'younger' than the cycle of the recipient.[1, 7, 23] The most successful combinations are achieved by arranging for the developmental stage of the embryo and the mother's cycle to be identical, or for the embryo to be slightly in advance of the recipient's uterine development. In farm animals, transfers are usually synchronous.

In most of the published reports on embryo transfer in animals surgery was used to place embryos in the oviduct or in the uterine lumen through the uterine wall. High rates of successful implantation have been attained: 75% or more of the transferred embryos implant in agricultural species[26, 28, 31, 32] and it has been reported that up to 90% of the embryos develop in laboratory species, although the figure is usually lower than this.[10, 27] If transfers were made through the uterine cervix, fewer demands would be made on the recipient, because surgery and perhaps even an anaesthetic would not be used. This method has been called inovulation[3] but at first it achieved a dubious reputation because it reportedly gave low rates of implantation in several species. Recent work on mice and cattle has changed the situation. Interest grew when successful transfer through the cervix was reported in cattle,[37] and implantation rates of 20% or more were later obtained.[30] More recently still, embryo transfer through the cervix in cattle has become much more successful and simple, with almost 50% of the transferred foetuses developing well past implantation or to full-term.[39] Improvements in embryo transfer through the cervix have also been reported in mice, with a success rate equal to or greater than that of surgical transfer.[24] Several hundred foetuses have now been obtained by this procedure and the results might be improved if the present use of anaesthetics could be discontinued. Preliminary studies with radio-opaque markers[33] have shown that this approach could be successful in women, for small amounts of culture medium can be placed in the desired position in the uterine cavity.

FOETAL GROWTH AFTER TRANSFER

The number of offspring produced from embryo transfer varies with the species. Considerable numbers have been obtained in laboratory animals—300 or more foetuses in some studies. By now, the number of mouse offspring resulting from transfer after both fertilization and embryonic culture *in vitro* must run into several hundreds, and several thousands after *in vivo* fertilization, *in vitro* embryo culture and then transfer. In rabbits, the figures are about 50 and several hundred, respectively. In farm animals, fertilization *in vitro* has not been successful, although embryos recovered as such have been cultured for up to three days before transfer. The number of foetuses or offspring in these species must now run into several hundreds each. No work has been reported on non-human primates because the development of the necessary techniques for recovering oocytes or for fertilization *in vitro* has so far proved very difficult.

All the evidence obtained from transfers has consistently pointed to one conclusion: there are no induced anomalies attributable in any manner whatsoever to the culture and transfer of embryos. Neither has there been any indication of an increase in the incidence of malformations of any kind in these species. Rates of implantation were sometimes low compared with natural mating, but improved techniques in mice, sheep and other species have now reduced the difference to small proportions. When factors such as the disturbance of the recipient by the operation, the loss of embryos during transfer and endocrine deficiencies in the recipient are taken into account, the frequency of implantation appears to be close to that found after natural mating. Other evidence confirms that the risks of abnormal development after embryo culture are very low. The preimplantation embryo is highly resistant to teratogenic agents (for reviews, see refs. 2, 5, 9, 18, 40 and 41). Alkylation, freezing and warming, irradiation with X-rays and treatment of the embryos *in vivo* or *in vitro* with toxins, antibodies, viruses and many other agents have not resulted in any confirmed increase in anomalies over control values. The few reports of induced anomalies have been negated by further work.

These observations stand in stark contrast to the effects obtained if embryos receive such treatment *after* implantation, for at this time many agents can induce anomalies. Two reasons offered for the difference between preimplantation and postimplantation embryos are that the preimplantation embryo can repopulate its tissues from the few undamaged cells which escaped the effects of the teratogen, and secondly that its cells are resistant because they are undifferentiated. Why undifferentiated cells are more resistant to teratogens is not clear.

Preimplantation embryos in the process of cleaving show no tendency to develop abnormally as a result of direct manipulation. Preimplantation embryos are astonishingly labile and can survive extensive dissection and treatments such as the destruction of one or more cells of the cleaving embryo, fusion of two or more embryos, the disaggregation and reaggregation of blastomeres, withdrawal of large quantities of cytoplasm and nuclei, removal of trophoblastic cells, and being turned inside out. The frequency of implantation is high after these treatments, and the overwhelming majority of embryos differentiate normally. These observations confirm the extensive data on this extreme resistance to induced damage.[19, 22, 25, 38]

CHROMOSOMAL IMBALANCE IN EMBRYOS

A possible exception to these observations concerns the induction of chromosomal anomalies. Preimplantation embryos can tolerate wide changes in their chromosomal constitution and still cleave normally, but most of them die after implantation. Dispermic fertilization, or the inclusion of the polar body chromosomes in the egg, can lead to triploidy, and errors in the movement of chromosomes on these spindles could lead to trisomy (the presence of one extra chromosome, as in Downs' syndrome [mongolism]). A small proportion of trisomic human embryos can develop to full term, although it is doubtful whether any human triploids have survived.

Triploidy could arise through delayed fertilization but has not been found in human embryos cleaving *in vitro*. Trisomy is a remote possibility, and its origins must be considered. Anomalies in the inheritance of the sex chromosomes can be traced back to the testis or the ovary,[29] whereas trisomies for the autosomal chromosomes apparently originate in the ovary because their incidence is closely related to maternal age.[6, 17, 18] Chromosomal errors could occur in three stages of growth of the oocytes: in early stages when the oocyte is in the foetal ovary (that is, prophase of meiosis—I), during the long resting stage between birth and adulthood (dictyotene) and during the final stage of growth of the oocytes (diakinesis to fertilization). Anomalies during each of these three phases have been held responsible for the induction of trisomy. Events during either of the first two periods have no relevance whatsoever to work on fertilization *in vitro* and embryo transfer. The cause of trisomy during the final period has been ascribed to factors such as delayed fertilization or viral infections, which are postulated to disrupt the ordered segregation of chromosomes in the egg. The theories on delayed fertilization[20] in older married couples have not been accepted, and evidence in animals shows that delayed fertilization does not lead to trisomy.[18] Nor have the data on viruses withstood further analyses.[18] Trisomy is thus unlikely to stem from fertilization *in vitro* or the culture of embryos, and triploids evidently do not originate in culture. Nevertheless, amniocentesis and the culture of foetal amniotic cells after about 14 weeks of gestation must be used to examine human foetuses resulting from embryo transfer for trisomy and triploidy.

TRANSFER OF HUMAN EMBRYOS

Advances in methods for the collection of preovulatory human oocytes, their fertilization *in vitro* and the cleavage of embryos *in vitro* could help many infertile couples to have their own children. The methods of oocyte collection have been outlined:[34] various hormones are given to the patient in order to control the growth of the oocytes and the changes leading towards ovulation; shortly before ovulation is expected, the oocytes are collected by laparoscopy, a simple surgical method which makes minimal demands on the patient. Oocytes collected in this way can be fertilized with spermatozoa collected from the husband, and the embryos will develop in culture through several cleavage divisions.[15, 16] In this way, embryos are available at stages where they would normally enter the human uterus, thereby raising the possibility of the transfer of human embryos. The embryos can, if necessary, be cultured beyond the stage at which they can be transferred, for several of them have been grown to expanding blastocysts,[36] which is the stage of attachment to the human uterus during implantation. The cleavage of embryos has been watched closely and has been shown to be regular: the nuclei have been normal, differentiation of the embryos has followed an ordered pattern, and various observations have been made on early human development. Chromosome counts on 15 embryos showed none that were triploid, although the exact chromosome number was difficult to identify because of the very few mitoses available for study.

Sporadic reports have appeared about embryo transfer in women, but no successful implantation has been formally claimed. Transfers could almost certainly be done non-surgically through the cervix and should present no difficulty. Infections should be easily controlled and the fine catheters necessary to traverse the cervix and uterus should cause no tissue damage. To begin with, transfers would probably be made with 8- or 16-celled embryos in order to conform with natural events. Examination of the uteri of patients given hormones showed that suitable stimulation was achieved for implantation, although hormonal supplements may be needed during the early stages of foetal growth. Cleaving embryos are obtained after laparoscopy from slightly more than half the patients,[16] and recent work implies that laparoscopy could be avoided in those patients who failed to respond sufficiently to the hormones.

Successful embryo transfer would alleviate the childlessness of many couples. At a conservative estimate 20 000 married women in the U.K. have tubal occlusion and perhaps six or seven times this number in the U.S.A. Other forms of infertility could also be cured, for example 'unexplained' infertility, and too few spermatozoa. Demands on the patient are not excessive, for hormone injections and laparoscopy, while not pleasurable experiences, are very mild forms of treatment and surgery. Laparoscopy is now a routine part of investigations into infertility and other illnesses, and the treatment does not damage tissues. The cost of the treatment is not high, nor is the necessary organization too complicated. Most infertile couples in the U.K., from almost any walk of life, would probably be able to afford this treatment if they had to undertake it privately. Surgery takes considerably less than 30 minutes, the patient needs to stay in hospital for two or three nights at most, and the costs of media and apparatus for embryo transfer are very small when apportioned between patients. Many patients are likely to be in their thirties, having tried other methods to overcome their infertility, and difficulties might arise with them because the incidence of infertility rises with maternal age even in women without any known lesions.

Some of the comments that are made about the wider implications of embryo transfer appear to be irrelevant or misleading. Debates on the imminence of genetic engineering, for example, are highly imaginative. The spectre of cloning is often raised, although no adult offspring have yet been produced after nuclear transfer in any species, even *Xenopus*. Excessive concern over the 'camel's nose' argument, namely that a series of small advances leads to the acceptance of all possible applications, so that cloning must follow from embryo transfer, seems unworthy of serious consideration. Likewise, suggestions that the infertile should not be cured because of the problems of overpopulation must be dismissed as mistaken. Adopting this suggestion would lead to changes in the doctor–patient relationship and would demand that an unfortunate minority be penalized for the sake of the majority. The only potential cause for concern for a long time to come appears to be the use of 'host' mothers for the convenience of an embryo donor, a practice that will require consideration should embryo transfer become established. We have defined our attitudes to the social, ethical and moral problems involved in this work.[12-14, 35] The great human benefit that could be gained stimulates us to continue our work with the full understanding and cooperation of our patients. We are sure that these studies will enhance the understanding of the basis of human conception and may provide valuable data on new clinical approaches to other human problems. We believe that our studies conform with the Hippocratic Oath in that they are for the benefit of patients and not for their hurt or for any wrong—indeed we believe they hold out the prospect of widespread benefit.

References

1   ADAMS, C. E. (1962) Studies on prenatal mortality in the rabbit, *Oryctolagus cuniculus*: the effect of transferring varying numbers of eggs. *Journal of Endocrinology* **24**, 471–490
2   AUSTIN, C. R. (1973) Paper given to the Committee on Ethics and Biology, British Association for the Advancement of Science, in press
3   BEATTY, R. A. (1951) Transplantation of mouse eggs. *Nature (London)* **168**, 995
4   BLANDAU, R. J. (1972) *The Use of Primates in Research on Human Reproduction (W.H.O. Symposium)*, Karolinska Institute, Stockholm
5   BRENT, R. L. (1970) in *Congenital Malformations* (Proceedings of the Third International Conference, The Hague 1969) (Clarke Fraser, F. & McKusick, V. A., eds.), pp. 187–195, Excerpta Medica, Amsterdam, ICS 204
6   CARR, D. H. (1971) Chromosomes in abortion. *Advances in Human Genetics* **2**, 201–257
7   CHANG, M. C. (1950) Development and fate of transferred rabbit ova or blastocysts in relation to ovulation time of recipients. *Journal of Experimental Zoology* **114**, 197–225
8   CHANG, M. C. & PICKWORTH, S. (1969) in *The Mammalian Oviduct*, University of Chicago Press, Chicago
9   DEGENHARDT, K. H. & KLEINEBRECHT, J. (1971) in *Intrinsic and Extrinsic Factors in Early Mammalian Development (Schering Symposium)*, Advances in the Biosciences, vol. 6, pp. 547 & 556, Pergamon, London
10 DICKMANN, Z. & NOYES, R. W. (1960) The fate of ova transferred into the uterus of the rat. *Journal of Reproduction and Fertility* **1**, 197–212
11 DZIUK, P. J. (1969) in *The Mammalian Oviduct*, University of Chicago Press, Chicago
12 EDWARDS, R. G. (1971) in *The Social Impact of Modern Biology*, Routledge & Kegan Paul, London
13 EDWARDS, R. G. (1973) Fertilization of human eggs *in vitro*: morals, ethics and the law. *Quarterly Reviews of Biology*, in press
14 EDWARDS, R. G. & SHARPE, D. J. (1971) Social values and research in human embryology. *Nature (London)* **231**, 87–91
15 EDWARDS, R. G., BAVISTER, B. D. & STEPTOE, P. C. (1959) Early stages of fertilization *in vitro* of human oocytes matured *in vitro*. *Nature (London)* **221**, 632–635
16 EDWARDS, R. G., STEPTOE, P. C. & PURDY, J. M. (1970) Fertilization and cleavage *in vitro* of preovulatory human oocytes. *Nature (London)* **227**, 1307–1309
17 FOWLER, R. E. & EDWARDS, R. G. (1970) in *Modern Trends in Human Genetics*, Butterworths, London
18 FOWLER, R. E. & EDWARDS, R. G. (1973) The genetics of early human development. *Progress in Medical Genetics* **9**, 49–112
19 GARDNER, R. L. (1971) in *Intrinsic and Extrinsic Factors in Early Mammalian Development (Schering Symposium, Venice)*, Advances in the Biosciences, vol. 6, p. 279, Pergamon, London
20 GERMAN, J. (1968) Mongolism, delayed fertilization and human sexual behaviour. *Nature (London)* **217**, 516–518

[21] HEAPE, W. (1890) Preliminary note on the transplantation and growth of mammalian ova within a uterine foster mother. *Proceedings of the Royal Society of London (B Biological Sciences)* **48**, 457–458

[22] LIN, T. P. (1969) Microsurgery of inner cell mass of mouse blastocysts. *Nature (London)* **222**, 480–481

[23] McLAREN, A. & MICHIE, D. (1956) Transfer of fertilised mouse eggs to uterine foster mothers. I. Factors affecting the implantation and survival of native and transferred eggs. *Journal of Experimental Biology* **33**, 394–416

[24] MARKS, S., THEORELL, M. & LARSSON, K. S. (1971) Transfer of blastocysts as applied in experimental teratology. *Nature (London)* **234**, 358–359

[25] MINTZ, B. (1965) in *Preimplantation Stages of Pregnancy (Ciba Foundation Symposium)*, Churchill, London

[26] MOORE, N. W. (1968) The survival and development of fertilized eggs transferred between Border Leicester and Merino ewes. *Australian Journal of Agricultural Research* **19**, 295–302

[27] MOUSTAFA, L. A. & BRINSTER, R. L. (1972) The fate of transferred cells in mouse blastocysts *in vitro*. *Journal of Experimental Zoology* **181**, 181–192

[28] POPE, C. E. & DAY, B. N. (1970) Cleavage and survival of swine ova cultured *in vitro*. *Journal of Animal Science* **31**, 1035

[29] RACE, R. R. & SANGER, R. (1969) Xg and sex-chromosome abnormalities. *British Medical Bulletin* **25**, 99–103

[30] ROWSON, L. E. A. & MOOR, R. M. (1966) Non-surgical transfer of cow eggs. *Journal of Reproduction and Fertility* **11**, 311–312

[31] ROWSON, L. E. A., MOOR, R. M. & LAWSON, R. A. S. (1969) Fertility following egg transfer in the cow: effect of method, medium and synchronization of oestrus. *Journal of Reproduction and Fertility* **18**, 517

[32] ROWSON, L. E. A., LAWSON, R. A. S. & MOOR, R. M. (1971) Production of twins in cattle by egg transfer. *Journal of Reproduction and Fertility* **25**, 261–268

[33] STEPTOE, P. C. (1973) *Proceedings of the VII World Congress on Fertility and Sterility*, Tokyo, 1971, Excerpta Medica, Amsterdam, ICS 278, in press

[34] STEPTOE, P. C. & EDWARDS, R. G. (1970) Laparoscopic recovery of preovulatory human oocytes after priming of ovaries with gonadotrophins. *Lancet* **1**, 683–689

[35] STEPTOE, P. C. & EDWARDS, R. G. (1972) The research of today and the ethics of tomorrow, B.M.A. Scientific Meeting, Southampton. *British Medical Journal* **3**, 342–343

[36] STEPTOE, P. C., EDWARDS, R. G. & PURDY, J. M. (1971) Human blastocysts grown in culture. *Nature (London)* **229**, 132

[37] SUGIE, T. (1965) Successful transfer of a fertilized bovine egg by non-surgical techniques. *Journal of Reproduction and Fertility* **10**, 197–201

[38] TARKOWSKI, A. K. (1970) Germ cells in natural and experimental chimeras in mammals. *Philosophical Transactions of the Royal Society of London (Series B Biological Sciences)* **259**, 107–112

[39] TESTART, J. & LEGLISE, P.-C. (1971) Transplantation d'oeufs divisés, chez la vache, par voie transvaginale. *Comptes Rendus Hebdomadaires des Séances de l'Académie des Sciences, Série D Sciences Naturelles (Paris)* **272**, 2591–2592

[40] TUCHMANN-DUPLESSIS, H. (1969) in *Foetal Autonomy (Ciba Foundation Symposium)*, Churchill, London

[41] WILSON, J. G. (1965) in *Teratology: Principles and Techniques*, University of Chicago Press, Chicago

Biological roots of the human individual

MASSIMO PIATTELLI-PALMARINI*

Of the five 'characters' in the A.I.D. drama (i.e. the mother, the donor, the stepfather, the child and the doctor), the one most easily released from ethical predicaments on the basis of biological considerations is the doctor.

In 1958 Gurdon[1] clearly demonstrated that in amphibians each cell has a full complement of genetic material which can give rise to a complete replica of the entire organism. Although experimental evidence is limited to aquatic frogs few biologists doubt that this applies to humans. Therefore, each living cell, whether part of the epithelial tissue, the liver, the brain or any other organ, presumably contains an invariant complete genotype. In this respect the germ cell is not different from the rest.

Referring to ethical problems relating to abortion, François Jacob[2] recently wrote that life never starts; life continues and a fertilized egg is no 'more' alive than a spermatozoon or an unfertilized egg. If it helps us to refer to 'potential human beings', then we might regard all cells of our bodies as potential copies of ourselves and even a mild scratch as leading to the loss and destruction of thousands of complete genome packets. However, the legitimacy of the very concept of a 'potential human being' is questionable. I propose to redefine this concept in terms of a complementarity between biological and social endowments. If we acknowledge that the 'conception' of a new human individual is a social act, the claim that a set of partially differentiated cells is a potential human being is no more legitimate than the claim of the letter cluster *gawagay* to be a potentially meaningful word in the English language. Thus, having acquitted the doctor of the charge of injuring potential human beings, we can leave to his conscience the problem of how to deal with already existing human beings and evaluate the risks of the artificial insemination he is performing, as he would with other surgical interventions.

* I wish to thank Professor Fried for discussions out of which the ideas for this paper arose.

Let us now see whether the biological and anthropological sciences can relieve the other characters in the drama of their predicaments.

SOCIAL AND BIOLOGICAL MEANING OF CONCEPTION

Historically, man as a biological entity originates as the result of freely chosen sexual intercourse between a male and a female of the human species, this intercourse leading to adequate physiological satisfaction and accomplishment, at least on the part of the male partner. The subsequent stage of development at which the dignity of a full human being is bestowed on the developing embryo is still subject to debate. The Catholic tradition has unhesitatingly endowed the fertilized egg with an everlasting soul, thus equating the material constitution of a new genome with all the prerequisites for immortality. Nowadays, the assumption implicit in the legalization of abortion is that a set of more or less differentiated cells is far from being a human person, and that this status can only be conferred upon the future individual by the parents-to-be when they fully accept their ensuing responsibilities as parents and educators. Just as they were free to have intercourse or not, with or without contraceptive devices, so they are also free either to allow the new individual to develop fully or to remove it early enough for the survival or health of the pregnant woman to be unaffected. In many animal species the moment of physical separation between mother and baby at birth undoubtedly marks the beginning of a new individual history. In humans it represents a major discontinuity in some of the embryological processes of maturation, but it is far from being the end of dependence on the mother. The newborn human infant is not autonomous and without prolonged and competent care over several years is unable to survive. The ethical issue is to determine the exact point in biological development and growth at which the commitment of the mother to accept and care for the infant is irreversible. This point is far from being well defined biologically and can only be established on a largely conventional basis.

The formation of a human individual therefore depends on free and willing intercourse, awareness and acceptance of pregnancy, attachment to and care of the infant after birth, and continuity in the process by which the child becomes independent of its mother and father at both the physical and the emotional level. The absence of any one of these stages impairs the full development of a new human being. It is interesting that in traditional Catholic doctrine the only occasion on which abortion is accepted is after rape, when the woman has the moral right to use mild measures, although not to damage her own body tissues, in attempting to expel the consequences of an unwanted fertilization.

That is, mutual assent is still accepted as a necessary prerequisite for the pro-creation of a new human being.

The biological and ethical issues concerning abortion, child care, attachment, education and affective relationships between parents and offspring are well known. However, many factors underlie the making of a human personality and any sharp division between biology and culture, between scientific knowledge and social considerations, would be arbitrary. The whole concept of a person and his existential 'feeling-in-the-world' depends as much on the history of how he came into being and on awareness of all the bonds linking him with nature and his fellow men as it does on his having a healthy body and a well-balanced mind.

Two aspects of this generative process can be isolated: (a) the conscious acceptance of pregnancy and its practical consequences up to the moment of birth as a major modification of the psycho-biological state of a woman. Accordingly the developing embryo is in all respects an extension of the mother's body, to which it belongs. (b) Mainly after birth, the developing organism is a new entity which becomes progressively independent and which is destined finally to have full independence.

It is difficult to disentangle these two aspects and to define the rights of the mother as opposed to those of the child. A major practical consideration is that a newborn baby can be entrusted to a woman other than the biological mother for maternal care. This possibility of surrogate nurture tightens the bonds to society as a whole, while making the connection with the mother less biological and more psycho-affective. Ethology shows that for most mammals, including monkeys and some apes, an infant can only be accepted by a female who has just undergone parturition, and in some cases acceptance can only take place within a critical period lasting a few hours. However, the late Daniel Lehrman showed[4] that, if their circulating systems are connected during late pregnancy and parturition, a pregnant rat can transmit to a virgin animal the hormones needed to induce her to build a nest and accept and care for the newborn pro-geny of the other animal. This shows that the hormonal 'storm' induced by pregnancy and parturition is a sufficient and necessary trigger of the maternal response. In humans, this is far from being apparent, although there are indica-tions that endocrinological factors influence attachment and maternal care. By all biological, psychological and affective standards, therefore, adoption cannot be regarded as a fully adequate substitute for maternity. This consideration is particularly relevant to the egg transfer techniques recently developed by Edwards and Steptoe.

Implantation of a fertilized egg into the uterus thus has no new significance for the genesis of the individual at a basic biological level, provided that the genome or genetic make-up of the embryo is derived from the gametes of the known mother and father. But if the sperm donor is unknown, or if both the sperm and the egg donor are unknown, the abnormal genesis of the individual poses some embarrassing questions.

Here the rights of a woman to accomplish fully her biosocial role clash with the rights of the person who is being brought into existence. Any consideration of one at the expense of the other must be closely examined. Professor Fried (pp. 41–45) will be developing detailed arguments against eugenic abuses and here I shall merely investigate a few complementary considerations about possible excessive randomization in gene pools leading to a genotype without a history. The production of stereotyped individuals is a dreadful perspective, which Huxley's *Brave New World* effectively dramatized, but indiscriminate randomness is in my view no less dangerous. I firmly believe that sperm banks, egg banks and test-tube fertilization should be avoided.

HEREDITY AND RANDOMNESS

The concepts of inheritance and genetic continuity were developed mainly for socio-economic reasons concerning legal rights and the transfer of land and material goods. In agricultural societies the individual is the recipient at birth of a constellation of rights, obligations and a shared destiny. In hunter–gatherer societies the newborn is automatically endowed with group or tribe exclusions issuing from kinship structures. The mere fact of being the son or daughter of a given person determines forever the restricted range of choices for subsequent marriage and reproduction. Genes are destiny in archaic societies. (In hierarchically organized groups of apes, baboons, hamadryas, macaques, etc. where practically all babies and youngsters are the offspring of a single dominant male, the overthrow of the dominant male and his replacement by a successor quite commonly leads to babies and very young adolescents being exterminated with the active aid of their mothers. It is as if the genetic domination of the new dominant male was reinforced by the group through physical destruction of the old strain.)

In contrast, bourgeois civilization is fluid, and from its beginnings has assumed that man is the product of his education. Nature counts for virtually zero, culture for almost everything. The oscillating moods between an aristocratic, sometimes racist, gene-bound conception of mankind and a pan-culturalist view of the newborn baby as wax to be imprinted generates an ambiguity towards the genetic history of the individual in present-day western society. Genetics are invoked only in cases of extreme misfortune such as when successive generations of a family have organic diseases, physical malformations or schizophrenia, or conversely whenever a conspicuous fortune or a kingdom is at stake. In between, scant attention is paid to genetic history.

Recent evidence on monozygotic twins reared apart suggests that the influence of the genetic programme on behaviour and social adaptability is much more powerful than previously thought. Infectious diseases, mental illness, acquisitiveness and quantifiable intellectual performances bear the mark of genetic determinism. This is no cause for wonder to the biologist.

The awareness that each of us is a random assortment from maternal and paternal heritage, with a considerable addition of cultural conditioning, is ancient and universal. The famous anecdote referring to Isadora Duncan and Bernard Shaw reminds us of the essential impossibility of programming the outcome of our fertile matings. Paradoxically, even if we suppose that we are totally conditioned by our genes, we are reassured because nobody has intentionally arranged the genes the way they are. This randomness allows for genotypic uniqueness and non-responsibility on the part of the parents. When we choose a partner and entertain the idea of reproduction, we implicitly accept his or her genetic endowment as a suitable pool out of which molecular processes will blindly complement our respective genes to extract the blueprint of our descendants. One can be held responsible for a marriage and for the decision to have children at all, but beyond these decisions lies the no-man's land of autonomous biological chain reactions. Control is responsibility; where there is no control there can be no responsibility. But if we now admit (as biology indicates) that genetic determinism is crucial and that whatever perfection we can attain in education and parental care genetic influence will be decisive, the problem of whose genes we are lovingly caring for arises for test-tube babies. Anthropology shows that in some matrilinear societies where paternity is most uncertain or irrelevant the mother's brother is the natural educator; he happens to be the only certain genetic ascendant: some of one's own genes must be present in one's sister's offspring. Similarly, lineage and kinship relationships usually determine adoption if the true biological parents and next of kin die.

Genes have never been taken less seriously than in our society, although interest in ancestry and the perpetuation of biological endowments has usually been strong. Marriage is largely random in our society but until recently we were at least aware of who was sharing genes with whom and of a parental bonding which secured continuity and identity.

Random fertilization is a new facet in the history of mankind and I am convinced that it is a negative one. Several reflections on biology and anthropology lead me to advocate strongly that serious criticism is needed before we enter a new era of random genetic assortments at variance with all established notions of human dignity and freedom. We are not here 'beyond dignity and freedom', but down at their roots. The point is to detect the collapsing of the historical and biological web which constitutes the human person. Marxists like to stress that man is the nexus of social relations in which he is embedded. I suggest that we must examine the genotype from the point of view of history, whose use in this context can be as illuminating as it usually is in economic and political matters.

Each of us—whether normally educated in our family, adopted, or taken care of from an early age by an organization or the state—realizes that two human individuals of opposite sex decided to fuse in a free act of love to give rise to a new individual. Whether these individuals intentionally willed such an outcome is a matter of secondary importance. But when donors, who will remain forever unknown, deposit in a tube some genetic material that is subsequently shaken in another tube to yield a viable mixture which is then implanted into the uterus of a fostermother, it is a different kind of man we obtain, at least from a social and evolutionary perspective. Perhaps these individuals will enjoy a perfectly normal and rewarding life, but the risk of loss of identity must be considered. If the desire of a relatively disadvantaged sterile woman for a child is fulfilled in this way, the notion that we have of a human being is likely to change. I fully subscribe to the Kantian criterion that every human being should be treated as an end in himself. This is why I am hesitant about the possibilities of these new techniques. I suspect that, besides the possible effects on the donor and the stepfather, we must consider whether the very person thus created is also merely a means for gratifying a frustrated maternity. Test-tubes can produce viable organisms but the machinery itself is an obstacle to the accomplishment of the very operation it triggers. The concept of a human individual includes both his genetic and his socio-cultural history and this appears to me as a positive acquisition of our civilization. The risk of biological manipulations is that they will destroy this delicate balance of nature and culture when they exceed the limits of bearable surgical interventions, and that they grossly contradict all our previous conceptions about the place of man in his time and his society. The prospects that have been envisaged of some biological manipulations of the human organism, such as hibernation, cloning and random genotype assortment, can only cause legitimate disquiet.

Hibernation entails the risk that living relics of the past will irrupt into a world which is not theirs and which will soon reject them. Cloning will perhaps one day reproduce individuals by the hundred, without considering that an individual has to be unique to be what he is. Finally, random gene assortment will produce test-tube babies who have a carrier but no mother in the genetic sense. Biology is a noble venture of the human spirit and whenever it also alleviates suffering its nobility can only increase. But it must proceed tentatively when it bears on such a sensitive matter. It took nearly three million years for the human species to attain a reasonable degree of coherence and we are still very far from a perfect balance between nurture and nature.

Pasternak wrote 'Rare are those to whom life discloses the undertakings which concern them: being overabsorbed by her deeds, upon enactment, she only allows for communication with those who wish her the best of success and who love her assets' (quoted by Jakobson[3]). Life has a wisdom which is far from having been exhaustively explored. The little we know seems to exclude the possibility that test-tube babies are those rare and fortunate beings to whom we shall be able to explain satisfactorily what undertakings we (and not life) intended for them.

References

[1] GURDON, J. B., ELSDALE, T. R. & FISCHBERG, M. (1958) Sexually mature individuals of *Xenopus laevis* from the transplantation of single somatic nuclei. *Nature (London)* **182**, 64–65
[2] JACOB, F. (1972) *Le Monde*, 19–20 November 1972
[3] JAKOBSON, R. (1971) *Poétique*, no. 7, p. 316
[4] LEHRMAN, D. S. (1961) Hormonal regulation of parental behavior in birds and infrahuman mammals in *Sex and Internal Secretions*, (Young, W. C., ed.), Williams & Wilkins, Baltimore, and (1971) personal communication.

Discussion: biological aspects

Stallworthy: When you said that A.I.D. is done only when the husband is infertile, did you mean that it *should* be done only when the husband is infertile?

McLaren: According to the literature it is only performed when the husband is infertile or suffers from a severe genetic disease. Most practitioners who write about the circumstances in which A.I.D. could or should be done dismiss the possibility of using it for unmarried women or when the husband either has not given his consent or is fertile.

Stallworthy: A recent article[21] seemed to suggest that A.I.D. was used in that particular clinic as a primary method of treating infertility even before an investigation had been carried out, and that only when it failed was the patient properly investigated. If this trend is developing, the sooner it is discussed the better.

McLaren: It seems extraordinary that A.I.D. should be used before the husband's semen has been examined.

Mason: The article may have been misinterpreted. I don't know of anybody using A.I.D. as a treatment, except when the husband has azoospermia. When the male is completely lacking in spermatozoa, the woman need not be examined by laparoscopy if she appears to be normally fertile before A.I.D. is attempted. If she fails to conceive within three months, then more extensive investigations could be made. The article did not mean that A.I.D. is used as a treatment to see whether the patient conceives.

Stallworthy: Investigation of the male, biologically and clinically, has not developed to anything like the extent that investigation of the female has. We must have a greater basis of understanding when we accept a male as the donor.

Parkes: Apparent male infertility can cover a wide range of conditions, from sub-fertility to absolute sterility. Unless A.I.D. is restricted to cases of absolute sterility, when there is no possible hope of periods of relative fertility occurring, it seems to me that if intercourse between the husband and wife is continued while A.I.D. is being practised it is always possible that the husband is the father of the child.

McLaren: Cases of relative infertility tend to be treated by A.I.H. For instance, when only a few motile sperm are present in the husband's semen, these can be collected, stored and concentrated before being used in A.I.H.; then pregnancy sometimes results. In general, doctors reckon that a virtual absence of motile sperm is an indication of infertility but, as you say, obviously there is a small and finite chance that the husband will be the father.

J. H. Edwards: Although our studies of infertile men (who had, we were assured, potentially normal wives) are limited, we found that sperm is an extremely unreliable indicator of fertility in several ways. Of the 1% of marriages in which the infertility was due to the husband, I doubt if more than 10% of the husbands would be found to be infertile on reexamination. One examination gives an assessment of vigour and quantity on that occasion only; even virtual absence of sperm can be temporary. More important, quantity gives no idea of the quality. Only bull's semen is routinely examined by electron microscopy. A testicular biopsy often shows chromosomal derangements which are not revealed by visual inspection. If A.I.D. is going to be used on grounds of male sterility, there simply is no realistic way of assessing more than a small minority of infertile males as truly infertile.

Kilbrandon: But if the man and his wife have had sexual intercourse together for many years without pregnancy, there is at least a circumstantial probability of some infertility.

J. H. Edwards: I think most infertile couples survive investigation without anything being discovered.

Piattelli-Palmarini: Why is artificial insemination available only to those who specifically ask for it and not suggested to patients?

McLaren: Presumably because the ethical and legal basis of A.I.D. is uncertain at present.

Mason: To suggest A.I.D. just after telling the husband that he is sterile is not a good idea. Some months, at least, should elapse before the couple start A.I.D.; they must adjust to the shock. Then if they return enquiring about their suitability for artificial insemination one can discuss it.

Philipp: I was asked by the Regional Board to start an A.I.D. service in our hospital. Some of the problems we had may be relevant to our discussion. First, I said I would not start it unless the Regional Board or the Department of Health took all legal responsibility for it. They replied that my medical defence union should take the responsibility. I disagreed, and after I had scrutinized a document they sent me that dealt with some of the matters mentioned by Dr

McLaren, I concluded that no decision had been made about the legality or illegality of A.I.D., about its possible failure or the consequences of complications. I was still concerned that we might be sued in ten years' time because, for example, a child had a mental defect. After the Department of Health had said they would take full legal responsibility, we decided to set up a clinic.

Next came the matter of getting donors; we first chose medical students who were affiliated to a London teaching hospital. However one of the conditions binding these students at the hospital was that they could not be used for any clinical or experimental purposes. So, we now have one of our doctors running a private A.I.D. service. We were told that we could not pay the donors for National Health Service patients because that would set a precedent; if we paid donors for semen, we ought to pay donors for blood transfusions. In our Harley Street practice, we can pay the donors, but cannot charge for the practice of A.I.D., which is a ridiculous state of affairs. It is semi-clandestine. Even if this symposium does no more than issue a statement about the moral, legal and ethical situations for the guidance of departments of infertility, a great service will have been rendered.

One example of the sort of infertility which we have to investigate is a man who had been so injured that semen was not able to pass through his ducts, although his testicular biopsy was satisfactory. Such biopsies prove either that, if the testes are making sperm, the ducts are blocked or that sperm is not being formed. If this latter finding is coupled with a history of mumps, for example, we have reasonable grounds for supposing that the man is sterile. We want more than a small chance that A.I.D. will work on any occasion, but we are illogical enough to advise the couple to have intercourse too, for there is a minute chance that the husband might fertilize his wife. This is to salve their consciences, if either has qualms about this.

Himmelweit: If A.I.D. is not very likely to be successful on the first occasion it is used, how sure can the woman be that the semen she receives later is from the same donor, since it is apparently the doctor who finds a suitable but anonymous donor?

McLaren: The woman is given no information about the donor, who may be different each time. Some practitioners of A.I.D., particularly in the U.S.A., use a mixture of semen, in which case there would be no possibility of knowing who the donor was.

Stone: How far does the medical practitioner satisfy himself that the semen is from the reputed donor? You said that in this country the medical practitioner likes to know the donor, Dr McLaren. At a symposium reported in the *American Practitioner*[1] it was suggested that the donor should deliver the semen at a different door from that used by patients. If the sperm is not produced on the premises there could be substitution, as Professor Himmelweit implied. Does the doctor insist that the semen is produced in the surgery or is it delivered?

Mason: In my practice, the donors bring the specimen to me personally. Many produce it on the premises, because this gives better samples and results; we put the semen straight into the incubator and use it, if possible, within an hour. One must know and trust one's donor. One of my prejudices against banks of frozen semen is the possibility of an error in the labelling of the specimen. The practitioner must have this process under his own control and must take the responsibility.

Kilbrandon: What is on the label on the specimen?

Mason: We usually put the donor's christian name.

Kilbrandon: Why use a name at all, especially if the semen is all mixed together?

Mason: That is not my practice. We try to match the characteristics of the husband with those of the donor. Of course, this is not possible in great detail, but we try to match height and colour of hair, for example.

Himmelweit: I am surprised that the matching is primarily with regard to external appearance. Do you not attempt some genetic compatibility in much the same way as an adoption society carefully evaluates the characteristics of the true parents and attempts to match these with those of the adoptive parents?

Mason: We do investigate. First, the donors must be perfectly fit and healthy. We now enquire about illnesses in their families among uncles, aunts, brothers, cousins, parents and grandparents. For example, before you marry, you do not ask your partner if his grandmother had diabetes, whereas if our potential donor's grandmother had diabetes, he would not be a donor. We also ask ourselves what sort of person the donor is. We require them to be above average in intelligence. I feel that I can give a more intelligent donor to a less intelligent patient, but not the other way round—perhaps I am wrong.

Since most of our donors are introduced by other donors, we know something about them beforehand and learn more over the period that they come in to deliver the samples. Having got to know him as a person, we do then have to make some judgement. Nobody can be God; but certainly if we believe that the donor is unsuitable, we reject him. As regards actually matching the donor to the couple we always consult the couples. A minority have extensive wishes such as musicality, athleticism etc., which we can often match. When we cannot, we discuss the matter with the couples.

J. H. Edwards: Adoption should not be in any way regarded as a good example to follow. My experience of adoption has been unfortunate. On being asked to advise about adoption, I found that casually taken pedigrees discriminated, particularly on vague grounds, against some couples who wished to adopt. Any robust, large family probably has a diabetic and a schizophrenic, so to some extent the question is whether the person comes from a vigorous, healthy family which is sufficiently numerous and close to know of such events. A grandmother who develops diabetes in her sixties is no basis for unsuitability; but a diabetic donor or even a donor with a diabetic brother might be a more serious matter. The casually taken pedigree history merely excludes honest people with good memories. Adoption is not a useful precedent because the basis for adoption was established before it was clear that such hereditary diseases as exist in man are either extremely rare or chromosomal in nature (and detectable or recessive). I agree that pedigrees can be useful for a few obvious diseases such as haemophilia. Simple genetic tests should be done, as obviously they were in Dr Mason's clinic for rhesus-negative patients. I presume you examine the haemoglobin in Jamaican donors, for example?

Mason: Yes, we would examine them for sickle cell trait.

J. H. Edwards: The analogy of bulls' pedigrees is extremely unsatisfactory, because there only dominant genes are detectable, and these are rare in man; the other genes are so complicated that the family history is going to be virtually useless. Clearly people with many criminal offences or obvious disorders are not desirable, but from the technical aspect a genetic expert would have no particular advantage over an intelligent general practitioner in choosing a suitable donor; the exotic rarities which can be transmitted are rare and often not detectable.

Kilbrandon: Most of us when we get married take our chance on genetic history. I see no reason why we should not do the same with A.I.D.

Stone: There is even less likelihood that this kind of enquiry into genetic history takes place before every act of sexual intercourse between persons who are not married to each other. Why should we worry that it is not done in this very small percentage of cases?

Piattelli-Palmarini: The ethical question is not only one of personal motivations in the abstract but relates to men and women, because women respond specifically to a cultural code which has been forced onto them. It is considered that a woman may only attain fulfilment as a female being by bearing a child. At the same time she is psychologically forced to submit to surgical (or at any rate mechanical) interventions as the only expedient by which an alien seed can be introduced into the marital nexus, if the woman is fertile but the husband is not and the couple want a child. Why should the insemination be artificial? Why is it not acceptable that she might have a baby from another person by natural insemination? This channelling of the woman's needs and the way in which she may accomplish these needs through a male morality deserves more attention.

Stone: Many women seem to feel this great social pressure on them to have a child. A visitor to this country from the United States gave evidence in November 1972 to the Select Committee of the House of Lords on discrimination against women in employment. According to her the American experience has been that a large programme of education in contraception or abortion is not needed to reduce the birth rate. All that is needed is to reduce the social pressure on people to have children. This seems to be one reason for the recent rapid decline in the birth rate in the U.S. Is this whole phenomenon the result of pressures brought on women, namely that the one way in which a woman can justify her existence on this earth is by producing a child, preferably male?

Mason: I don't think so. The people who come to infertility clinics certainly do not come merely from pressure by other people. They are desperate to have babies. The social pressure is much less now. Since contraceptive advice has been available, I have seen the almost worrying change in attitudes of girls in this country: in complete contrast to the situation ten years ago, many girls say they do not want to have a family now or even ever.

Steptoe: The women who come to fertility or infertility clinics have thought very carefully. They will be responsible parents; probably much more so than many of the couples who have a high percentage of unplanned and unwanted pregnancies.

Stallworthy: The idea that the mother who has borne a child, whether through artificial or natural insemination or even embryo transfer, necessarily wants a child badly may be an oversimplification. Doctors know full well that some women, having conceived as a result of any method, then want to destroy the child by abortion. They have satisfied some inner desire to prove to themselves that they could conceive and having done so that is an end to the matter. This is a rare situation—but it does happen.

Piattelli-Palmarini: If an A.I.D. child developed a disease of unknown aetiology, would those in charge of a sperm bank reveal any family history of disease?

Mason: We have had one such case: a baby with spina bifida. The doctors concerned wrote asking for information, and we gave them as much as we could. We even arranged for the donor's spine to be X-rayed.

Piattelli-Palmarini: Has one the right to store any information about the child to which he will have no access?

Mason: In general, A.I.D. children do not know that they were born as a result of this technique, so it is unlikely that the request would come from the child himself.

McLaren: In one case,[8] a 17-year-old boy became disturbed when the man he believed to be his biological father died of a hereditary illness. The boy was anxious that he himself might develop the disease in later life. When the doctor who had performed the insemination explained the nature of the conception, the boy was not only relieved but grateful to his 'stepfather' for having had the foresight to take this action.

R. G. Edwards: Dr Piattelli-Palmarini seemed to be concerned about the effect on the offspring of learning that he was an A.I.D. child. Surely pertinent observations must have been made in many other situations, such as bastardy or where the wife has had extramarital relations which were later revealed, and the effects of these influences must be documented in the literature. The only difference is that the A.I.D. child exists because of the deliberate decision of the father and mother. Does this deliberateness worry you, or do you think it would worry the child?

Piattelli-Palmarini: When the child already exists, the fosterparents can try to solve the problem. With A.I.D., the child was not there; the problem did not exist. The parents deliberately created both the person and the problem. The A.I.D. child's origin, his or her coming into existence, is different. I wonder about his feeling of identity.

R. G. Edwards: Do you mean we must look for an element in A.I.D. not present in adoption or bastardy?

Steptoe: And are you suggesting that an infant conceived in love has some special genetic privilege?

Piattelli-Palmarini: A special problem exists where the biological father is unknown; it is not that the fruit of love is genetically different but that other children have a history whereas an A.I.D. child has no history. In the genotype of people procreated normally the element of indeterminacy is balanced against determinacy. The resulting concept of 'self' harmonizes with a feeling of identity, which may be discordant or absent in A.I.D. children.

Graham: Problems of identity are likely to arise much later on in life, at adolescence. It is interesting that A.I.D. children do not generally know that they are born as a result of this particular method of conception, because the risk that they will find out is always considerable. It is now regarded as good practice for adopted children to be told about their adoption as early as they can possibly understand that they are not the biological but the social product of their adoptive parents. How do A.I.D. parents cope with this situation?

The whole question of identification in personality development is complex. Children, both consciously and unconsciously, take on parental characteristics, and conscious modelling is partly based on the child's belief that he is the genetic as well as the social product of his parents. For A.I.D. children, that is not true.

I believe that adoption is a reasonable parallel, though there are obvious differences. Dr Edwards has suggested that we should be able to compare the psychological effects of children born in different sorts of circumstances with those born from A.I.D., but the literature is complex and the published results differ greatly. Some workers suggest that adopted children, for example, have a considerably higher rate of psychological disturbances; others that they do not. In my opinion, they do not have a much higher rate of psychological disturbances unless adopted late after an unsettled early life. What is most important is their domestic background.

It should be possible to investigate whether, as Dr McLaren suggested, the children born from A.I.D. have normal intelligence. I doubt whether the intelligence of the children is likely to be affected. The particular objection that was raised in the Japanese studies[17] (p. 5) seems invalid, for one could easily control for social class.

Adopted children who suffer disturbances do fantasize about their biological parents. These fantasies are important in the nature of the disturbances they manifest. In A.I.D., another element is introduced into the situation. The fantasies are likely to be modified by the knowledge that the father is not the genetic father. It will not be long before psychological disturbances are being attributed to A.I.D., perhaps mistakenly, but certainly the fantasies of people who are born in this way are going to be different from those of adopted children and of children reared by their biological parents.

Some factors, such as the severity of behavioural and emotional disturbances in childhood, are measurable. Investigations of adopted children have met with great difficulties. Adoption agencies are reluctant to hand over information, as they are naturally concerned about the confidentiality of their information. Will it be possible to conduct a scientific investigation? There are arguments for and against: for example the intrusion into privacy, the possibility of upsetting well-adapted individuals and so on. We need to know more before we can decide whether the law should make known its opinion on this issue. It cannot do so without sufficient scientific information.

Kilbrandon: Clearly A.I.D. and adoption have this in common: in time a child will discover that his father is not his father. The great difference that we may have to consider is that in adoption, a child *can* discover who his real parents were. (This is more difficult in England than it is in Scotland, but it can be done.) Whether there should be some machinery by which the child can discover who its donor was is a different question.

Steptoe: Might we not be overtaken by events? It will be difficult to set up a prospective study, because in England a large number of people are unable to adopt owing to the lack of babies, and the situation is deteriorating month by month. I believe A.I.D. will have to become more widely used in the alleviation of the problem of infertile couples.

Feilding: The use of mixed semen in A.I.D. must complicate the two situations we have considered: fantasies with respect to parenthood entertained by the progeny of these unions and the scientific determination of their genetic heredity. Are the variations in practice between countries and clinics known? Where the donor is known, is a record kept, by whom, and who has access to it?

Stallworthy: The pattern is not standard in the U.K. at the moment. A subcommittee of the scientific advisory committee of the British Medical Association, under the chairmanship of Sir John Peel, is investigating the problems of banks of fresh or frozen semen and related topics.* At present there are not many centres where artificial insemination from a donor is practised on a large scale, but to my own knowledge the practice varies from place to place.

Mason: I do not know anybody who is mixing semen in England.

Stone: Dr Piattelli-Palmarini, you said that in matrilineal societies paternity was uncertain, because sexual intercourse by the women was absolutely unrestrained. Are you saying that this happens in all matrilineal societies or just in a few? Anthropologists have told me that although lawyers and others like to talk about primitive societies in which everyone was promiscuous, this was just another golden age that never existed. Research shows that there never was such a society, and that the evolution of society has seen not the imposition of more rules, but rather a lessening in the number of rules.

Piattelli-Palmarini: Some societies where paternity is known or reasonably certain are so structured that everyone lives in his or their mother's dwellings. The child's mother and maternal uncle therefore happen to share the same roof. In other societies mating is relatively free (even though several taboos and prohibitions still exist). Then, the father being unknown, the child is entrusted to the maternal uncle for education and training in several skills.

I wished to stress that adoption through random assignment of fosterparents or conception through random fertilization is a unique facet of present-day societies. However, I am sure that no anthropologist would admit that a society or tribe can exist without some rules governing mating and marriage. Kinship structures appear to be the minimum prerequisite for a society. For the anthropologist the elimination of all kinship and parenthood structures would be equivalent to the elimination of matter itself for the physicist or the geneticist.[10]

Dunstan: It has been mentioned that Gurdon et al.[14] showed that it was possible to transplant nuclei from intestinal cells to ova in *Xenopus* without impairing their ability to bring about normal development. Has this experiment been repeated for human cells?

Piattelli-Palmarini: To my knowledge it has never been attempted because

* *Note added in proof:* The report has been published: (1973) Report of panel on human artificial insemination. *British Medical Journal* **2** (Suppl.), 3–5

human eggs cannot be manipulated to the same degree as the large eggs of *Xenopus*.

R. G. Edwards: No one has yet taken a nucleus from an adult amphibian of any species and produced an adult offspring from it. In other words, the experiment which has been an important part of all the debates on genetic engineering has not yet been fully accomplished even in amphibians. It might be feasible, but all the results so far show that when a nucleus is taken from an adult cell and placed in an egg, many of the offspring will die as larvae—or at least soon after hatching, even if the nucleus is passaged twice or more through egg cytoplasm (e.g. ref. 13). Metamorphosis occurs in a very few cases. Their work has not been done in the human species. The few experiments in mammals, such as the mouse, have shown that the embryos grow abortively, and it now seems doubtful that the transferred nucleus is incorporated into the embryo.[4, 11]

Piattelli-Palmarini: Do you agree that the genetic information is there?

R. G. Edwards: In general I do, provided genetic information is defined clearly. The success of cloning varies greatly with the species. In certain species of *Rana* development was much retarded in comparison with that found in *Xenopus*, although this is now questioned.[22]

Piattelli-Palmarini: Gurdon's aquatic frogs (*Xenopus laevis*), which were of parthenogenetic origin, were obtained through transplantation of a nucleus from an intestinal cell into an unfertilized enucleated egg of the same animal.[14] The rate of success of this manipulation is about 1%. Dr Edwards is right, this relatively low rate of success drops to zero if one performs this operation in an adult frog. This experiment has yet to be done in tadpoles, although one can take tadpoles in a well-advanced stage of development. The historical debate between Wilhem Roux, who claimed to have demonstrated a loss of genes during differentiation, and Hans Driesch, who obtained complete animals from cleaved embryos, has ended with Driesch in the right: Gurdon has shown, beyond any reasonable doubt, that each cell of an individual has a complete genome.[14] Differentiation is not loss but selective repression of genes. Although this has not yet been proved in mammals, it is unlikely to be otherwise.

Fried: Dr Edwards, is your hesitation about the full complement of genetic material in every cell of a human body a prudent scientific doubt in the sense that, until it has been demonstrated, you are not going to make that assumption? The history of science is too full of things which are so in principle and turn out not to be so; that is how progress is made.

Is there a similarly negative or futuristic aspect to parthenogenesis? If cloning is not possible, can the same results be obtained by manipulating the egg so that it splits and turns into an embryo?

R. G. Edwards: My doubts about the success of cloning are concerned mainly with the production of identical viable offspring. Possibly somatic mutations in the donor nucleus and changes in the organization of genetic material might occur during differentiation. In mammals, maternal intrauterine effects could also modify foetal characteristics. The use of a donor nucleus to code for a complete and identical embryo has still to be proved, although it might be possible. I do not doubt for one moment that all or most of the genetic informations is potentially present in each cell.

Parthenogenesis of eggs has been induced in various mammalian species; rodent embryos can grow to advanced stages of differentiation.[25] This was surprising, for much debate has stressed the lethal potentiality of homozygosity for some mutants. Newborn parthenogenones are presumably possible, especially if such mouse foetuses can proceed to almost half-way through gestation. I do not see any close relationship between this success with parthenogenesis and cloning, since the technical problems are different. Biologically, parthenogenesis involves some of the genetic material present in the egg in the first place. Such a method would be pointless clinically, since its advantages are highly dubious, and there is no means of controlling the genetic information retained in the egg.

Williams: Dr Edwards, you confined your remarks to the transplantation of the woman's own ovum or embryo, saying that that was the sole objective of your work. Was this an ethical or a biological remark? Is it technically possible to transfer an embryo between women?

R. G. Edwards: Biologically, there is no problem; it would be far easier to transfer an embryo to another woman, because we would not have to induce ovulation in the recipient by means of exogenous hormones, and would thus establish better conditions for pregnancy. Our doubts are largely ethical.

Bevis: Embryo transfer is utterly different from artificial insemination in that we are taking the husband and wife and not the wife and a third person.

Williams: Embryo transfer was said not to raise the same problem as A.I.D., because there is no donor. But that is like saying that A.I.H. does not raise the same problems as A.I.D. Any introduction of a donor raises similar problems. With two donors, as would be possible with embryo transfer, I believe the situation is easier, because it is simply very early adoption.

R. G. Edwards: In our paper we were describing our situation at the present time. I fully accept the point. Embryo donors would seem to be rare because the chance of a young woman lacking active ovaries is much smaller than that of a man having no spermatozoa.

Stone: Recently, the press reported an ovary transplant in South America. Is this something that should be taken seriously?

Steptoe: A young woman of 25 who had had most of her ovaries removed received a whole ovary, transplanted with proper anastomosis of blood vessels and removal of the remnants of her ovaries. She is now three months pregnant. This situation, in which a woman has a normal uterus and normal tubes but no ovaries (or ovaries which are not capable of functioning) must be extremely rare. No one yet knows what the outcome of this will be. It will be interesting, particularly if hormone support was necessary.

Parkes: Delayed fertilization is said to increase the probability of the result of a fertilization being female. What is the current view of this?

McLaren: Claims that the sex ratio of the progeny is altered by inseminating at different times in the cycle[2, 12, 15, 18] have been made but as far as I know none of this work has been repeated and confirmed.

Parkes: Could the abnormalities which can arise from delayed fertilization (pp. 5, 14, 15) result from fertilization of a stale egg by a fresh spermatozoon or of a fresh egg by a stale spermatozoon?

McLaren: Chromosomal abnormalities may result from fertilization of stale eggs, both in animals[3] and in man.[16] Use of stale sperm might have led to the death of embryos in some cases, and certainly to reduced fertilizing capacity,[20] but as far as I know not to any identifiable defects.

Parkes: You said that the lifespan of the human sperm in the female reproductive tract was short. How is the lifespan of sperm estimated?

McLaren: In animals, the fertile life of sperm has been worked out from the results of timed inseminations after ovulation had been induced with hormones at a known time. Apart from bats, which can store sperm in the female reproductive tract for several months, a life of 24–48 hours is usually quoted.[23] Much longer estimates are sometimes given for human sperm, but little reliance can be placed on these in view of the difficulty of knowing the time of ovulation. Motility of sperm recovered from the reproductive tract is a poor guide to fertilizing power.

R. G. Edwards: I agree, but Croxatto *et al.*[7] occasionally found that intercourse several days before the expected time of ovulation, which was fairly well known from hormone assays and recordings of body temperature, had resulted in conception. In certain cases, therefore, human spermatozoa can live for a long time in the female tract; certainly they can live for days *in vitro*.

Parkes: Another complication in humans is that the apparent intervals between insemination and the expected time of ovulation might sometimes be in error because of coitus-accelerated ovulation.[24]

Stallworthy: We have washed spermatozoa that appear to be histologically normal and active from the human uterus as long as three days after the last intercourse.

If, on delayed fertilization, the chance of a female developing were greater than normal, would a higher incidence of chromosomal abnormality be expected in the developing foetus? If that were so, and if the other 'ifs' were correct, one would expect to find an increased incidence of abnormality in the female rather than in the male.

R. G. Edwards: This is an interesting suggestion but I know of no relevant data. The best population to study would be Catholics using the 'safe' method of birth control, where according to some reports the number of anomalies is fairly high, as would be expected. Whether females displayed more anomalies than males has not been recorded.

Perutz: What are the present technical chances of sex determination in sperm, that is, of separating XX and XY sperm?

Parkes: That follows from my question about the possibility that delayed fertilization increases the probability of a female being produced. I am enough of a feminist to refuse to believe that a female is merely the product of a stale egg! If the possibility is substantiated, the only explanation I would accept is that some form of selection between X and Y sperm is taking place as they become older. This would imply that X spermatozoa (the female-determining ones) have a slightly greater stamina in the female tract.

Deliberate sex determination by separation of X and Y sperm has not yet been achieved, even in experimental animals, despite much work.

R. G. Edwards: Many people have tried to separate spermatozoa with different phenotypes, including various other classes besides those carrying an X or Y chromosome. If we could find a system whereby individual spermatozoa expressed their own characteristics, we could hope to separate X and Y spermatozoa. The one clear example of an increased rate of fertilization by spermatozoa of a particular type is found in mice,[6] and also positive evidence for the expression of transplantation antigens on spermatozoa and their segregation according to the type of spermatozoa has been claimed.[9, 26] Jílek & Veselský[19] question these observations, and it appears that some of the results were accidental and due to contamination. I believe that the only possible method of separating sperm is to find density differences in spermatozoa with X or Y chromosome, but no such differences have been reported that I am aware of. Recent work[5] has shown that two classes of rabbit spermatozoa, respectively carrying a haploid and diploid component of chromosomes, can be partially separated by centrifugation in a dextran density gradient.

Parkes: One can distinguish sperm by density differentiation, but the separation does not appear to follow the chromosomal composition.

References

[1] *American Practitioner* (1947) **1**, 227
[2] ASDELL, S. A. (1927) Time of conception and of ovulation in relation to the menstrual cycle. *Journal of the American Medical Association* **89**, 509–511

[3]   AUSTIN, C. R. (1967) Chromosome deterioration in ageing eggs of the rabbit. *Nature (London)* **213**, 1018–1019

[4]   BARANSKA, W. & KOPROWSKI, H. (1970) Fusion of unfertilised mouse eggs with somatic cells. *Journal of Experimental Zoology* **174**, 1–14

[5]   BEATTY, R. A. & FECHHEIMER, N. S. (1972) Diploid spermatozoa in rabbit semen and their experimental separation from haploid spermatozoa. *Biology of Reproduction* **7**, 267–277

[6]   BRADEN, A. W. H. (1958) Influence of time of mating on the segregation ratio of alleles at the T locus in the house mouse. *Nature (London)* **181**, 786–787

[7]   CROXATTO, H. B., DIAZ, S., FUENTEALBA, B., CROXATTO, H. D., CARRILLO, D. & FABRES, C. (1972) Studies on the duration of egg transport in the human oviduct. I. The time interval between ovulation and egg recovery from the uterus in normal women. *Fertility and Sterility* **23**, 447–458

[8]   ENNIS, J. (1972) A.I.D.: the gift of life. *Nova*, January issue, pp. 20–22

[9]   FELLOUS, M. & DAUSSET, J. (1970) Probable haploid expression of HL-A antigens on human spermatozoa. *Nature (London)* **225**, 191–193

[10] GODELIER, M. (1973) Discussion with Jacques Monod in *The Unity of Man* (Morin, E. & Piattelli-Palmarini, M., eds.), Editions du Seuil, Paris, in press

[11] GRAHAM, C. F. (1969) The fusion of cells with one and two-celled mouse embryos in *Heterospecific Genome Interaction (Wistar Institute Symposium Monograph No. 9)* (Defendi, V., ed.), pp. 19–35. Wistar Institute Press

[12] GUERRERO, R. (1970) Sex ratio: a statistical association with the type and time of insemination in the menstrual cycle. *International Journal of Fertility* **15**, 221–225

[13] GURDON, J. B. & LASKEY, R. A. (1970) The transplantation of nuclei from single cultured cells into enucleate frogs' eggs. *Journal of Embryology and Experimental Morphology* **24**, 227–248

[14] GURDON, J. B., ELSDALE, T. R. & FISCHBERG, M. (1958) Sexually mature individuals of *Xenopus laevis* from the transplantation of single somatic nuclei. *Nature (London)* **182**, 64–65

[15] HAMMOND, J. (1934) The fertilization of rabbit ova in relation to time. *Journal of Experimental Biology* **11**, 140–161

[16] IFFY, L. (1963) The time of conception in pathological gestations. *Proceedings of the Royal Society of Medicine* **56**, 1098–1100

[17] IIZUKA, R., SAWADA, Y., NISHINA, N. & OHI, M. (1968) The physical and mental development of children born following artificial insemination. *International Journal of Fertility* **13**, 24–32

[18] JAMES, W. H. (1971) Cycle day of insemination, coital rate, and sex ratio. *Lancet* **1**, 112–114

[19] JÍLEK, F. & VESELSKÝ, L. (1972) The occurrence of lymphocyte antigens in boar spermatozoa. *Journal of Reproduction and Fertility* **31**, 295–298

[20] KOEFOED-JOHNSEN, H. H., PAVLOK, A. & FULKA, J. (1971) The influence of the ageing of rabbit spermatozoa *in vitro* on fertilizing capacity and embryonic mortality. *Journal of Reproduction and Fertility* **26**, 351–356

[21] MASON, B. A. (1971) An alternative to adoption (an interview). *World Medical Journal* **7**, 24–25

[22] MUGGLETON-HARRIS, A. L. & PEZZELLA, K. (1972) The ability of the lens cell nucleus to promote complete embryonic development through to metamorphosis and its applications to ophthalmic gerontology. *Experimental Gerontology* **7**, 427

[23] RESTALL, B. J. (1967) The biochemical and physiological relationships between the gametes and the female reproductive tract. *Advances in Reproductive Physiology* **2**, 181–212

[24] SINGER, I. & SINGER, J. (1972) Periodicity of sexual desire in relation to time of ovulation in women. *Journal of Biosocial Science* **4**, 471

[25] TARKOWSKI, A. K., WITKOWSKA, A. & NOWICKA, J. (1970) Experimental parthenogenesis in the mouse. *Nature (London)* **226**, 162–165

[26] VOJTÍŠKOVÁ, M., POLÁČKOVÁ, M. & POKORNÁ, Z. (1969) Histocompatibility antigens on mouse spermatozoa. *Folia Biologica Praha* **15**, 322–332

Ethical issues in existing and emerging techniques for improving human fertility

CHARLES FRIED*

The existing and emerging techniques affecting human reproductive processes have been disturbing to scientists, legislators, judges and the public generally. This is particularly true for those techniques designed to enable otherwise infertile couples to have children, whether through the sperm of the male partner or not, or in some more advanced methods with the eggs of a donor female. Unease has demonstrated itself in the persistent embarrassment, if not unwillingness, about the incorporation into the legal system of norms that would give legitimate status to children conceived from donated genetic material. This unease has also shown itself in calls for legislation flatly prohibiting certain techniques and research projects, such as the suggestion before a committee of the United States Congress that experimentation with human eggs and particularly experiments leading to the cloning of human individuals should be severely limited. This unease and hesitancy has been criticized as obscurantist, muddle-headed, conservative and unreflecting.

I want to probe beneath the surface manifestations of that unease to see whether it is possible to state in a coherent and adequate way what values, if any, are affected by these new techniques, whether these values are endangered by some or any of these techniques, and what implications this analysis might have for research policy.

At the outset, I dismiss the argument that, given the present population crisis and given the existence of homeless children, the development of techniques for rendering fertile women who would otherwise be unfertile is a social nuisance to be discouraged at all costs. Dr Piattelli-Palmarini showed (p. 21) that the changes and development in the human female as a result of pregnancy and birth have a hormonal and thus a physiological basis. The desire for such condi-

---

* This paper owes much to discussions with Dr Piattelli-Palmarini.

tions and development therefore cannot be said to be merely a socially conditioned desire for something good. Moreover, as Dr Piattelli-Palmarini also implied, this hormonal change may lead to a more adequate mother–child attachment and thus is the basis for a network of far-ranging social links that might have important implications for social relations generally. Finally, such a fulfilment of human female nature is a valid objective for social effort, because given its basic quality it might be considered as a claim to basic human fulfilment, like the claims to education, decent housing, health care and so on.

Having acknowledged the value of this research and of the techniques emerging from it, we ask why is it rational to observe any cautions? Why should one suggest any restraints at all in procuring what resembles normal physiological pregnancy and birth? What is implicated is the integrity of the concept of the person as a unique entity, responsible not only to the society which nurtures and surrounds him, but in a sense carrying a responsibility to himself, to his own perceptions and choices, in short the notion of the individual as a centre of consciousness and self-determination. Is such a concept of the individual worth preserving? For one thing, it seems to have certain important positive implications, such as the capacity to resist social pressures, critically to oppose dominant ideologies and thus to display a sense of responsibility to self, to one's own perceptions and original intellectual concern. This feeling of irreducible uniqueness may be related to a concern for objective scientific truth as well as for creativity in general, simply because it implies resistance to a notion of scientific truth or artistic invention as something wholly conditioned by social needs or pressures.

Although this line of argument is obviously too speculative to be conclusive, it seems sufficient to point out that our concept of the human person is determined by the relation of that person to his own physical being, and by the history by which that physical nature has assumed the form which it has. If such demonstration can be made, then a firm basis has been laid for the otherwise apparently vague unease to which these developing techniques of manipulating human fertility have given rise, namely an unease about modifying the concept of the human person and thus the relations of people to each other and to themselves. It might be said that the human person, considered as a free and rational entity, believes himself to be only in part the product of the choices and pressures of the society to which he belongs. To some extent he believes himself to belong also to himself, to have a responsibility to himself, to be determined by things that are uniquely his own. Accordingly the sense of self-determination is part of a family of concepts that have to do with the sense of uniqueness and individuality. Because a particular human person is unique, as an individual, he is also self-determining, and his concept of self-determination comes from the fact that some of the things that determine his actions and beliefs are not the product of social actions, choices and pressures.

This sense of uniqueness and individuality importantly implicates one's own body, because the most palpably unique aspect of each individual is his physical individuality: the simple fact that he is not and knows that he is not exactly like other people. (Hence the problems and discomfitures about identical twins.) The concept of a unique, randomly assorted genotype (clearly demonstrated in modern genetics) gives this intuitive sense of uniqueness an objective physical basis. But this sense of individuality is related not only to uniqueness but to randomness, to the unpredictable materialization of that particular one out of a great many possibilities which both produces and expresses the uniqueness. These concepts converge to make up the notion of an individual as a 'self', who has not been totally programmed or fabricated, who is unique.

The more one's genetic basis, that is one's most intimate physical nature as an individual, is subject to manipulation, the less plausible it is for this individual to consider himself as a unique product which is not wholly and totally the result of choices and policies of others. The more his genetic nature is a result of the choices of others, the more he must consider himself as a social product, the result of a mechanism which may make more and more claims upon him.

The argument against significant affirmative manipulation of human genetic material (by affirmative I mean the choice of certain characteristics, as opposed to the effort to exclude a clear and precise range of negative characteristics) has so far been considered only from the point of view of the individual who would know himself to be the product of such manipulation. But of course the argument has a social dimension as well. The use of such techniques allows a vast and deep extension of the political power of those who would control the technique. Not only could they impress their values and preferences on the next generation through their eugenic choices, but this would be done in the most insidious possible form: the 'agents' of their policies would be agents not because of an argument or a philosophy they have been convinced of, not because the pressure of self-interest had been brought to bear on them, not even because they were being coerced into this agency, but because they were created to be the sort of person who would in their most intimate natures carry forward their agency. It is not as if these agents would somehow find it difficult to choose not to carry forward the agency, but rather that their very existence *is* that agency.

Presumably the refinement of technique that would be necessary to bring about such a futuristic situation is a long way away. But grosser *affirmative* eugenic manipulation is probably coming daily more within our grasp. Consider the position of the citizen in a commonwealth where some unspecified but significant proportion of the population is the result of eugenic choices. This society may be entirely democratic: one man—one vote. The unease a citizen would feel in such a situation, however, points out the significance that the concept of randomness has not only in our conception of ourselves, but in our notions of a democratic state. The notions of democracy are undermined in any society where rigidly propagandizing education of youth leads to an utterly predictable conformity among the resulting adults (who, for example, may then safely be left entirely 'free' as democratic citizens); the genetic programming of citizens would undercut even more the notion of the democratic commonwealth as a forum for citizens with free choice. Since both the propagandized and the programmed citizens would exercise a democratic franchise without any external constraints, our objection to this state of affairs shows that the concept of democracy implies not only absence of external constraint on the exercise of our democratic rights, but also freedom and openness in the process which leads us to be who we are and how we use our freedom. In the genetic arena this once again brings us to the importance of randomness as a value.

The above indicates how a highly developed eugenic programme might interfere with the concept of self, person and individuality. A more difficult question is why artificially assisted fertility, which respects total randomness when the donor eggs or sperm are chosen in a totally random way from pools of donors, would similarly undermine these central concepts. Piattelli-Palmarini has referred to the non-mental bases of such crucial relations as maternal affection and attachment. Moreover, one *is* heavily determined by the parental upbringing that one goes through in the first twelve years of life. A person knows himself to be largely the product of the parental love and nurture he has received. If parental love and nurture also have a correlate in the physical continuity of the genetic identity of the parents with this unique identity of the child, then both one's physical nature and the love one has received seem less contingent, more securely anchored in each other. The parents who love the child and support him are also the individuals who have provided him with his physical body, the people who have provided him with his unique genetic equipment; they are not utter strangers but those who have given him the necessary love and support which make him spiritually able to develop the humanity for which his body is a basis. Any sundering of this complementarity, of the physical and emotional continuity between parent and child, may lead to a corresponding strain on the sense of ease and confidence which the child feels both in this physical being and in his social relations, particularly in the family. The child from random eggs and random sperm grows up in a family situation which is in some sense wholly the result of chance, and this too may be a disturbing and unsettling fact.

Thus I suggest that the usual reproductive methods where those who care for the child also provide the genetic material, without however determining the whole nature of the child (in the sense that a vast quantity of randomness still enters into the genetic make-up), mean that the concept of the individual and his physical nature stands somewhere between wholly indeterminate randomness and complete determination by the choice of others. It is for this reason that the techniques under consideration have important repercussions on the concept of individuality. Undoubtedly, these repercussions and the associated values do not provide a basis for demarcation between the permissible and the impermissible. Scientists and physicians might, therefore, feel disturbed that all that has been produced are values and considerations to be taken into account, that no sharp line has been drawn with clear-cut prohibitions to be enacted relieving scientists of the need for choice. Rather, what emerges is the notion that the preferred objectives for medical research and techniques should be the assistance, first of all, of 'canonical' pregnancies, and secondly, of those which combine the genetic materials of the man *and* woman who will commit themselves to caring for the child, or failing that, those which use the genetic material of one or the other of the partners.

Moral and social issues arising from A.I.D.

G. R. DUNSTAN

For the purpose of this paper I shall assume that the practice of A.I.D. is discussable as a matter of personal morality for the husband and wife concerned and for the donor; of professional morality for the medical practitioner; and of such social importance as to be cognizable at law and to require the attention of legislators. At present discussion of the personal and professional morality of the practice, like the discussion of its scientific validity, is inhibited because the practice has developed in ways unforeseen and unprovided for by law, with the result that existing legal categories have had to be bent, and even actively misused, in order to accommodate its consequences. Because governments have been given by their electorates neither a clear mandate for legislation nor that degree of moral agreement upon which legislation would necessarily be based, new legal categories have not been enacted. My purpose, therefore, is to suggest, first, means by which this social and legal inhibition might be removed, in order that the practice may be more openly assessed both scientifically and morally.

In the U.K., the Feversham Committee reported in July 1960,[8] having been appointed in September 1958. It had been under pressure to recommend the prohibition of A.I.D. as an offence; it declined to do so, though it expressed severe disapproval of the practice, and the hope that it would diminish. It located the act within the legal category of 'liberties', which 'while not prohibited by law will receive no kind of support or encouragement from the law' (Chap. 10 para. 266)—so accepting a suggestion put to it in evidence submitted by a committee on behalf of the Church of England.[2] Its proposals for legislative reform touched almost exclusively on proceedings for nullity or divorce; it recommended no amendment of the laws relating to legitimacy or registration of birth. The result, as seen 13 years later, has been to allow the practice to grow—in the U.K. as elsewhere, though probably at a slower pace than in the U.S.A.—with the social and moral consequences aggravated by the adverse moral judgement on the practice and the consequent refusal to consider amendment of the law at its most critical point, where it affects the status of the child, in the matters of registration and legitimacy.

The Feversham Committee pronounced the child conceived by A.I.D. undoubtedly illegitimate. A strictly correct entry in the Register of Births would record no name for the father, and so testify to the illegitimacy on the certificate. The entering of the mother's husband's name as 'father', an offence in itself, obscures the illegitimacy but does not cancel it. The name of the true father, the donor, though known no doubt to the practitioner, is not disclosed, for a variety of compelling reasons.

The sum of all this is that moralism compromises truth: a judgement that the act ought not to be done, while it continues to be done, gives rise to an accumulating deceit upon society, both in records and in relationships. It also prevents the gathering, reporting and scientific study of the basic information necessary for a proper judgement upon the extent and consequences of the practice, and upon its ethics. It is odd, to say the least, that in an era in which genetic research is for the first time becoming scientifically and socially significant, we are increasing, rather than decreasing, the area of uncertainty between genetic identity and social identity. Some area of uncertainty is inevitable: it is perpetuated every time a child, begotten by a father other than the mother's husband, is nevertheless registered and brought up as a child of the marriage. In the centuries before adoption was formalized it was accepted that the two identities did not correspond. But social policy, represented for instance by the system which interlocks a register of adoptions with the register of births, would appear to be aimed at diminishing the uncertainty. Research interest and social interests alike require that public records be reliable: most genetic counselling, for instance, is conducted, not on the evidence of karyotyping, but on the assumption that reputed parents and grandparents are genetic parents and grandparents; if that assumption cannot safely be made, prediction becomes the more uncertain; if it is invalidly made, the consequences of an erroneous prediction could be serious.

It is, therefore, a matter for serious concern that a new medical practice, grounded upon scientific research and so upon the high value put on truth, should in fact result in, and to some extent require, deceit and uncertainty. The secrecy involved in A.I.D. obliges the practitioner, the husband and wife, and the donor to conspire together to deceive the child and society as to the child's true parentage, his genetic identity. Truth is violated; credibility is undermined; and this is a serious ethical matter.

It is commonly assumed that it is in the child's interest that he be deceived as to his true parentage. The assumption may be warranted: I have insufficient competence in child psychology to judge whether he would be seriously harmed by the truth, or at what age he might safely learn it. But the argument might go the other way, when one considers the risk of suspicion, or of accidental disclosure, or of the circumstances of his conception coming into issue in matrimonial or testamentary proceedings between those whom he has accounted to be his parents—such litigation has occurred.[4, 6, 12] The fact of his illegitimacy—if such it be—complicates the issue for him, as for society. In a suit concerning maintenance in 1968, the Supreme Court of California held that a child conceived by A.I.D. to a married woman with the knowledge and consent of her husband is the legitimate offspring of the marriage;[11] an intermediate appellate court in New York in 1963 had ruled to the contrary.[6] The Feversham Committee, by a majority, rejected the suggestion that an A.I.D. child, accepted by the husband into the family, should be deemed legitimate. 'Succession through blood descent', it argued in its Report (para. 163), 'is an important element of family life and as such is at the basis of our society'. Two members dissented from the judgement and the reasoning. The argument, indeed, must be thought to carry diminishing conviction in contemporary England. There may be good reasons for attaching the descent of titles of honour and of entailed hereditary estates to 'blood descent'; these, though important, are few and identifiable enough to be made a special case. There would seem to be no compelling reason why these interests should be the basis of general legislation.

The Legitimacy Acts of 1926 and 1959 have considerably eroded the concept of 'legitimacy' altogether, and subsequent legislation, civil and ecclesiastical, has considerably lessened the social and economic disabilities of the illegitimate child. The decision of the Supreme Court of California, cited above, and an enactment of the State of Oklahoma in 1967, authorizing the practice of A.I.D. and declaring its issue 'legitimate', violate what logic is left in the application of the concept, by extending 'legitimacy' to a child not genetically related to both its parents. It seems as though the concept is incapable of further extension while retaining any meaning; it is socially useless. As an instrument for the expression of moral approval or disapproval it is manifestly inept and unjust: the stigma ought not, in morals, to rest upon the illegitimate child but upon the parents who gave it birth; the epithet is improperly transferred.

The next step might well be, therefore, not to try to extend the concept of 'legitimacy' further, but to abolish it (Cameron & Webb[1] reached the same conclusion from a totally unrelated study of the law concerning illegitimate children). It could well be replaced by the concept of 'acceptance', or of 'approbation'; this would give the status of social 'filiation' to any child accepted into the family by husband and wife, however begotten and conceived, and assure to it all rights, privileges and duties attaching to that status. The register of filiation would record the social recognition of the child. A separate genetic register would record its genetic descent, on the model of the adoption register, and as such would be open to inspection only by those who could prove a just and compelling interest in its contents. (Insemination with mixed semen would be forbidden; it would also be unnecessary.) Such a provision—grossly over-simplified, of course, in this outline, but capable, I submit, of legal embodiment —would better serve the public interest in social identity; it would lessen the incitement to falsification and deceit which impugns the worth of the present registration; it would give reliable general data for genetic research and coun-selling; and—assuming that the practice of A.I.D. will continue, and possibly be extended—it would provide material for an objective assessment of the practice. This latter is a scientific and social necessity, if ever there was one, for the present enforcement of secrecy has the result that the published studies are those of the practitioners themselves.[9, 10, 15]

Having thus removed, at least notionally, the instrumental inducements to falsification and deceit, it should be easier to examine the moral and social issues more openly. To do this thoroughly would require that the whole ground covered by the Feversham Committee be worked over again, in the light of advanced scientific knowledge and medical technique, and of such consequences as have been, or can be, surveyed.

The claim of the wife of an infertile husband upon an available medical remedy for her childlessness is—understandably enough—said by the practi-tioners to be high. They are themselves sensitive to the risk of 'giving' a child to a pathological mother and they state that they try to avoid doing so—though their methods of assessment do not always find favour with psychiatrist commenta-tors. There are, nevertheless, ethical limits to the degree of that risk. Further-more, the strong desire of a well-balanced woman to bear her own child, while it may exert a strong claim to satisfaction by medical intervention, cannot exert an absolute claim: if it could be met only at the expense of invading unacceptably other interests in society, the principle of distributive justice would require that it be not met by this means; help should be sought for the woman in some other way.

Paramount among the 'other interests' are those of the A.I.D. child: an act of 'compassion' towards the would-be mother might result in an act of injustice to her child. An area of great uncertainty surrounds, for instance, the question of concealment or disclosure of the method of his conception. The paper by Piattelli-Palmarini (pp. 19–25) argues how important the matter is. Since the practitioners in A.I.D. appear to work to a code of ethics in which justification derives from beneficial consequence, it would seem to be morally imperative that they should promote authoritative studies in this field as a condition of the continuance or extension of their work.[3]

Another area of moral concern is the relation of A.I.D. to the integrity of the marital relation. It is here that A.I.D. presents itself chiefly as a question of what was called, at the beginning of this paper, personal morality; though it is here also that religious interest in the problem has most concentrated, and persons professing allegiance to particular churches or religious communities are under duty to pay regard, varying in degree, to the moral teachings of those bodies. The Roman Catholic Church has pronounced authoritatively against A.I.D. for the married woman as much as for the unmarried, in statements from the Holy Office in 1897 and from Pope Pius XII in 1949 and 1956.[5] Two bodies appointed by the then Archbishop of Canterbury, a Commission in 1948 and a Committee in 1960, expressed adverse judgements, though each body had one dissenting member.[2, 13] No Christian Church in the U.K. known to me has explicitly favoured the practice, and the judgement of Jewish Orthodoxy is hostile. Western culture as a whole, in fact, influenced not only by the Judaeo-Christian religion but also by the Graeco-Roman tradition of philosophy and law, has emphasized the nexus between the begetting and conception of children and the shared or common life of the marriage and the family. (The concept of 'legitimacy' and 'illegitimacy' was an instrument, morally inept but practically useful, in support of this nexus.) Where deviations were tolerated socially, they were bound up with other social institutions now discredited, like the existence of classes, as of slaves, or serfs, or social inferiors, implicitly excluded from the norms of human relationship. Within the tradition, the conception of a child by seed other than that of its mother's husband was possible only by means of sexual contact between the wife and the father, with all its emotional content and potential; and this was denounced as adulterous. Fertilization without the adulterous association was not discussed because it was not possible. The new knowledge and possibility, however, invite ethical judgements of two sorts. Persons who hold that the nexus between marriage and begetting is inescapable and exclusive (as orthodox Jewry and the magisterial Christian Churches teach) will repudiate A.I.D. even though the insemination does not involve the act of adultery: the seed of a donor other than the husband would be held to 'adulterate' the marriage as milk would be adulterated by water or sugar by sand—a semantic elision which has led Christian bodies to press for the legal proscription of A.I.D. as adulterous, pressure which lawyers, with their insistence on verbal precision, have rightly resisted. Those, on the other hand, whose concept of the nexus ends with the physical congress of husband and wife, and who regard the semen of a third party with detachment as a mere fertilizing agent whose product in conception imports nothing alien into the marriage relation, would feel free, for themselves, to accept A.I.D. as a remedy for the infertility of their marriage; though whether such a cerebral judgement does justice to the whole socio-psycho-physical reality of the problem is a question which requires close discussion in the light of that research to which the present cloak of secrecy is a severe impediment.

Similar considerations apply to the donor. There is, again, a regrettable ignorance and uncertainty about his motives, avowed and unavowed, about the effects of his action upon himself, in the long term and in the short term, and about his suitability, objectively considered, for the role of progenitor of a child to which he will remain for ever unrelated. The self-gratification inherent in the act of masturbation was itself for long suspect to moralists in the Judaeo-Christian tradition; and they would still say that the pleasure must be 'ordinate', that is to say ordered and proportionate to a proper end. The giving of semen for examination, or for assisted insemination of a wife, would now be considered as done for a proper end and therefore licit in Anglican moral theology (ref. 2, p. 18 and note); formal Roman Catholic discipline would still appear to forbid it (ref. 5, p. 6), although moral theologians are now quoted who would permit it.[7] It would be much harder to describe the action of the A.I.D. donor as licit also. The moral difficulty attends, not the pleasure, but the moral requirement that a man should take full responsibility for the offspring of his loins—a moral obligation not invalidated by acquiescence in the irresponsibility of fathers towards their bastard sons. To moralists for whom this requirement is paramount it is not enough that the donor will be assured that 'someone'—the host mother and her husband—will be responsible for his child: the responsibility is exclusively *his*, because of the moral relationship assumed to derive from, and to attend, paternity; to beget, without the possibility of a continuing father–child relationship, would be to withdraw biological potential from personal potential—to reverse the long process of evolution by which biological capacities have been humanized. In a defined sense, therefore, the donor's action, made possible by human science, is anti-human: it isolates biological potential from the human potential. (There are cultures, it is true, where an uncle, for example, and not the father, assumes responsibility with the mother for the upbringing of the child; but within the kinship reciprocity is assumed—the father is also an uncle himself, and so exercises 'paternal' responsibility for nephews of his own. The A.I.D. donor is, in this respect, a social isolate without continuing responsibility.) Moralists for whom the word 'love' serves as a master-key to ethical problems might counter this objection with the assertion that the opportunity to do 'a loving act', namely to provide a childless marriage with a child, over-rides all other considerations; but it must be said in reply that such an assertion begs many questions about the nature of the act performed, and about the nature and obligations of 'love'; in the moral tradition within which this paper is written, 'love' cannot oblige a man to perform what is, according to the analysis given above, a less than human act.

The question whether donors of semen should be paid or not has clear moral implications—in relation especially to motive—and even clearer scientific implications, highly relevant to medical practice. A London practitioner appearing on BBC television on 26 September 1972 said that she paid her donors, and that she estimated their genetic fitness by asking them questions about their parentage and medical history. Titmuss[14] has demonstrated the medical and economic inferiority of a transfusion service in which donations of blood are paid for: the financial reward encourages the indigent to conceal relevant facts in medical history, and so increases the supply of infected blood. By a parity of reasoning, payment of donors of semen, with no evidence of genetic suitability other than unverified assurances about parenthood and medical record, suggests the taking of highly unethical risks from which the patient to be inseminated, her husband and the child to be conceived might prove the victims. Reluctant as we are to extend statutory regulation of medical practice, a minimum requirement, if A.I.D. is to continue, should be either a legal prohibition of the payment of semen donors, or an authoritative act by the appropriate professional body to eliminate the payment as an unethical practice. The practitioner also remarked, incidentally, that while scientifically it was 'an old wives' tale' that babies conceived at a particular time in the months were more likely to be boys, she nevertheless inseminated at that time, and did achieve more boys than girls. It must be asked how such a statement, in a television broadcast, stands with the ethics of the use of scientific information in relation to clinical work, and—in view of the strong desire in some women to have boy babies—how it stands with the ethics of advertising in medical practice.

There are other questions related to the nexus between marriage and parenthood. On empirical grounds—the necessity of both father and mother figures in the child's upbringing—as well as *a priori*, it must judged unethical to give a child by A.I.D. to an unmarried woman. A combination of empirical and *a priori* arguments would also prohibit A.I.D. for a wife without the informed and deliberated consent of her husband. In the same category stands the question whether a fertile husband should give semen for the insemination of a woman other than his wife. Since one essential ingredient of marriage is the mutual and exclusive exchange of procreative powers, a husband may not morally give to a third party what he has covenanted to give exclusively to his wife. On the analogy of the waiving of a privilege vested in a spouse, it could be held that she might waive her exclusive right by consenting to his donation of semen for this purpose—but only if it were already established that the act itself is not *per se* a wrong: if it were (and a view has been indicated that so far as it is a less than human act it *is* a wrong) consent would not set it right.

This paper has been concerned only with the practice of A.I.D. as it has been brought within my notice by those undertaking it. It has not gone further to examine those extensions of the practice which are read about, whether in use or abuse: the storing of frozen human semen, for instance, for future impregnation, either on behalf of the donor himself who has been sterilized meanwhile, or for impersonal use in the controlled production of a number of children from seed selected because of its supposedly favourable genetic characteristics. The pattern of the argument set out above could be extended to cover such practices. The further the act of insemination is removed, for instance, from the personal union and common life of the donor and recipient of the seed, the further from the human and therefore the more suspect morally the practice would be. So far as breeding for 'desired' characteristics goes against that degree of randomness and diversification which the evolutionary process itself requires, it would call for rejection on genetic grounds as well. But that is to speculate beyond the present purpose.

A certain impatience may arise when intangible moral and metaphysical considerations of the sort advanced in this paper are set up, as cautions and perhaps as impediments, against the 'practical benefits' which science and medical technology can achieve: is this no more than the perennial attempt to shackle science and obstruct progress? But in dealing with man, two sorts of inheritance are in man's keeping. There is the genetic inheritance, properly studied by science, still evolving, and properly to be brought within the range of human manipulation so far as that can be done without violation either of the process or of other essential human interests. There is also another inheritance, transmitted not genetically but culturally, also evolving, and also to be improved if the right criteria for improvement can be established. (The Christian looks to the future for those criteria, rather than, as is often supposed, to the past.) Within the cultural inheritance stand that cluster of rational, moral, emotional and aesthetic capacities to which together we apply loosely the terms 'humanity' and 'humane'. It is the task of the moralist—though certainly not his alone—together with the scientist to concern himself with the relationship of the one inheritance to the other. Forceful attempts to advance the first *may* not threaten the second; but they may; and wisdom would suggest that the more far-reaching are the powers of manipulation conferred by the science, the more searching should be the joint scrutiny of the risk.

References

1 CAMERON, B. J. & WEBB, P. M. (1967) Illegitimacy in *Family Law: centenary essays*, Wellington, New Zealand

2 C.I.O. (1960) *Artificial Insemination by Donor: two contributions to a Christian judgment*, Church Information Office, London. (The publication contains also the personal evidence of the then Archbishop of Canterbury, who disagreed with the conclusion of the Committee which he had appointed.)

3 C.I.O. (1966) *Fatherless by Law?* App. 1, Publications relating to the psychological need of a child to know his own father, Church Information Office, London

4 COLEMAN, A. H. (1965) Artificial insemination heterologous and the illegitimate child. *Journal of the National Medical Association* 57, 331–332

5 C.T.S. (1960) *Artificial Insemination. Evidence on Behalf of the Catholic Body in England and Wales* (submitted to the Feversham Committee), Catholic Truth Society, London

6 CURRAN, W. J. (1968) Public health and the law: artificial insemination. *American Journal of Public Health* 58, 1460–1461

7 HÄRING, B. (1972) *Medical Ethics*, p. 92, St. Paul Publications, Slough

8 H.M.S.O. (1960) *Report of the Departmental Committee on Human Artificial Insemination*, H.M. Stationery Office, London, Cmnd. 1105

9 LANGER, G., LEMBERG, E. & SHARF, M. (1969) Artificial insemination. A study of 156 successful cases. *International Journal of Fertility* 14, 232–240

10 LEVIE, L. H. (1967) An enquiry into the psychological effects on parents of A.I. with donor semen. *Eugenics Review* 59, 97–101

11 PEOPLE v. SORENSEN (1968) 66 Cal. Rptr. 7, 437 P. 2d 495

12 ROSENBERG, A. H. (1968) Legal aspects of artificial insemination. *New England Journal of Medicine* 278, 552–554

13 S.P.C.K. (1948) *Artificial Human Insemination*, S.P.C.K., London

14 TITMUSS, R. M. (1971) *The Gift Relationship*, Allen & Unwin, London

15 WATTERS, W. W. & SOUSA-POZA, J. (1966) Psychiatric aspects of A. I. (D.). *Canadian Medical Association Journal* 95, 106–113

Discussion: moral, social and ethical issues

Andrejew: Canon Dunstan, why are you so strongly against paying semen donors?

Dunstan: A strong case stems by analogy from Titmuss's comparison[6] between the blood transfusion service of the U.S.A., where 90% of blood is paid for, and that of the U.K. where almost all of it is given free. Because of the money motive, it is the indigent—the drug addicts, the educationally handicapped, the Negro population and the prison population—who supply the bulk of America's blood. Since they have strong reasons for concealing facts in the blood history, the incidence of infected blood is very high; 15% of the blood is wasted, and even so there is much infection with hepatitis from transfused blood plasma. In economic and medical terms the paid service is grossly inferior to the voluntary one. I accept the conclusions for social policy which Titmuss draws from his study. Payment of semen donors must invite concealment of material facts in family history, and this, with no more screening than a conversation with the gynaecologist-inseminator, would put patients and their children at risk. The general case against commercial semen donation is even stronger than that against commercial blood donation.

Andrejew: One can avoid the problem of concealment by using 'professional' donors, whose personal histories are well documented.

Graham: In the U.K. blood is donated on an unpaid voluntary basis and a high standard of purity is maintained. Arguably this is more desirable, for it represents something positive that one section of the community does for another. But how relevant is this to the donation of semen? Blood can only be given once every three months or so, whereas semen can be given much more often.

Mason: I agree; I don't think the parallel between blood donation and semen donation is obvious. Our semen donors are people that we have come to know well over a period of time and have been previously specially selected. People are not ready at the moment to give their semen free, as we donate blood. Possibly in another 10–20 years people will feel that they are helping couples who cannot have babies. At the moment the person who writes to me saying 'I feel it my duty to be a donor' tends to be, in my opinion, odd. Certainly I have rejected the ones of this kind whom I have interviewed.

R. G. Edwards: I understand that some doctors keep a record of their semen donors and that many donors ask the doctor to keep track of the child, in case anything should go wrong with his affairs. Canon Dunstan, how do you see the duties of a donor once he has given semen for the purpose of insemination?

The situation concerning the duties of the semen donor is now being discussed in Germany in connection with the right of the child to know the identity of his biological father.[2] Some of the suggestions of the U.K. Law Commission on injuries to unborn children[7] may also be relevant to this discussion, since live offspring may be given the right to claim for damages inflicted before fertilization.

Dunstan: Ethically, my chief concern is with the gap between the act of begetting and the acceptance of responsibility for progeny. I can see that in the interest of the solidarity of family and the security of the child the donor must not again come into the child's life and therefore must be excluded from what I regard as the moral obligation and fulfilment of parenthood. The feeling of responsibility by some donors supports my case on the one hand but, on the other, the practical difficulties of intervention by the donor are enormous.

Williams: I do not wholly agree with the formulations of either of our speakers. The idea fundamental to A.I.D. seems to be a distinction between the genetic and the social father. This is not unthinkable, for it is realized, perhaps not absolutely, in certain human communities, as we have already heard (p. 52). Moreover, the Latin terms *genitor* and *pater* are perfectly capable of bearing this distinction. Some of Canon Dunstan's worries were based on first distinguishing and then confusing these two notions. He seemed to be concerned that the genetic father was not carrying out the responsibilities of the social father. The model for the genetic father then becomes the sailor with a girl in every port who goes around the world irresponsibly scattering his Maker's image, as the phrase goes. He asked, by implication, isn't the donor rather like that? The answer is no, not at all. The malice in the sailor's action consists in leaving the child without a social father. When the genetic father is providing the materials for the birth of a child within a relationship which contains the social father, the objection that the genetic father is neglecting his responsibilities cannot apply. The important question seems to concentrate on the relationships of the social father and the mother to the child, and not on the relationship of the donor to the child. Of course, it would be terribly disruptive if the genetic father became an interested party. It is neither moral nor commendable on his part to become interested in the outcome; the arrangements should be such that he cannot do so. Why is that supposed to be immoral? It is only so if you confuse the notion of the genetic father and the social father. Professor Fried raised the question of what happens if one separates these two, which is the question we ought to be asking and not what happens if they are then run together again (whereupon we do get into a muddle, I agree). In answering his own question, Fried suggested certain rather alarming and allegedly manipulative considerations. Some of his objections depended on the idea of positive eugenic interference. Now I regard that as an exceedingly different matter both biologically and morally, as Dr McLaren told us. There are all sorts of objections to eugenic selection which involve a concept of the person that raise the problem that Fried mentioned, but which do not seem to me to be entailed in the idea of A.I.D. as such. Why should these two ideas be necessarily linked morally or biologically?

The suggestion was made that a person's somatic identity must relate to his genetic origins, and because a person is a somatic identity in a sense, one cannot properly separate the social and the genetic elements, a separation which would occur under a general A.I.D. practice. The zoological proposition that throughout the animal kingdom genetic parents are concerned with their genetic offspring (which is probably false to a large extent) is not acceptable, since animals do not have the concept of genetic offspring. We may observe that they are looking after the genetic offspring, but as soon as there is a cultural self-consciousness which involves having concepts of offspring, parental responsibility, for example, the whole argument is on a totally different basis. No zoological evidence could possibly explain any of these points. The answer must be social and cultural.

I agree with Fried's metaphysical view about the nature of persons, that they are a somatic identity, but I am not sure what follows from that. Certainly it is true that to be a person requires a bodily identity, a past, a social setting and a set of social identifications. The claim that because a person must have a genetic history, genetic identifications must constitute his conscious identity, does not appear to follow.

The whole point of the discussion must be to distinguish, not to confuse, the roles of the genetic and the social father. What are the consequences of separating these? Once the eugenic issue has been distinguished, no sound argument has yet been propounded that the consequences of separating them are metaphysically damaging.

Fried: I did not mean to suggest that this notion of being a person is threatened in any particular case, but rather that if the practice of A.I.D. becomes either general or usual the concept of the person would change. Would your doubts still hold then?

Williams: I meant my comments in the light of general practice. Probably the concept of the person would change to some extent; it is somewhat different in a society where the social and genetic father are identified from that in a society where these are further apart. The change would not necessarily be more manipulative, evidently damaging or anti-humanistic.

Himmelweit: The adopted child is told, 'you existed and I chose you'. The A.I.D. child would be told, 'I chose to make you with this raw material'. I agree with Fried that it is not a matter of eugenic planning; in A.I.D. a choice of parent exists which does not exist with the adopted child. At some stage, an A.I.D. child who derives in part from a mixed sperm bank may be told that he is such a child (many arguments favour telling him; previously it was thought that an adopted child should never be told the truth, but now we advise the opposite). Then the A.I.D. child might justifiably say 'I was made differently'. Such a person might also ask why mixed sperm from a bank was used, or 'why did the doctor, or you, not choose one special donor?' This problem of feeling that the mother chose badly is highly specific to the A.I.D. child. The idea of 'being made or manufactured' may be present. There was once a suggestion that the sperm of the most brilliant minds of the century should be banked. This seems a perfectly logical and socially sensible conclusion: I am not approving of it, but I believe it is a logical step which must be considered. The idea that A.I.D. will operate without eugenic planning is totally unrealistic; it might be bad eugenic planning but it will operate at some private level.

Kilbrandon: The parents could say to the child, 'we *did* choose the best— unfortunately Beethoven wasn't on offer'.

Williams: I do not see how you can distinguish this from the attitude of the child who asks his mother why she did not choose a better husband.

Dunstan: Professor Williams and I have stated two clearly different views. Part of my concept of humanity attaches social responsibility to genetic parenthood, while he, I believe, deems this unnecessary.

Williams: So do a lot of tribes; I am not alone in this. That they always ascribe social responsibilities to genetic parenthood is a false statement about human beings.

Dunstan: I did not say always. Even though the uncle in certain matrilineal societies may not be bringing up his own children, he brings up others. If we are going to generalize, we do attach responsibility for nurture to the fact of begetting; the question of whether the children being brought up are our own or someone else's is secondary.

Isaacs: The fact that adopted children have an identity and a sense of identity, when they may have no knowledge whatsoever of their genetic identity, disproves this idea that all identity is genetic. A considerable part of the sense of identity must be psychological, having developed early before anybody could tell the child how he was conceived or from what he was procreated. Of course, the parental attitude to the child is important; any sense of guilt on the part of the parents because they have had to tell a lie seems to me to be important psychologically.

Piattelli-Palmarini: Impaired identity may influence social behaviour. Fried and I agree that in scientific enquiry or philosophy it is most desirable to possess the self-confidence to withstand different ideologies or ideas which are shared by others. This is or ought to be a common situation. A person must have an opinion of his own notwithstanding the shared opinion, and be willing and able to impose, or to struggle for, his own ideas. The A.I.D. child may develop in two extreme directions. In the first, his thoughts can be and have been determined genetically by the choice his parents made and for which he bears no responsibility. In the opposite case, the awareness that his thoughts and beliefs are different to those of his fellows and consciousness of his uniqueness may make him unable to fight for his own ideas, and, further, lead him to believe that his thoughts have no relevance to those of 'normal' people.

R. G. Edwards: In comparing genetic and social identity, none of the arguments about adoption seem to establish the primacy of genetic identity because an adopted child is raised in the home and social circumstances of the parents, a background almost certainly totally different to that which the adopted child would have had in his own family. Professor Williams' comments about social rather than genetic identity in tribal systems are not necessarily valid because it would be necessary to be sure that the capacity existed for the offspring to express their genetic diversity; similarly with most adopted children. Scientifically, we need a situation where children could be raised under common circumstances but their differences are encouraged. There we would see the effects of genetic and social identity.

Piattelli-Palmarini: More than a hundred monozygotic twins have been raised separately from each other, sometimes unaware of his existence, and yet the coincidence of infectious diseases, mental disorders and less obvious effects between each twin is amazing.[4, 5, 8]

Perutz: How are people so confident about knowing what produces a feeling of identity between parent and the child? Studying imprinting in ducks, Hess[3] showed that the identification of the duckling with the mother begins in the egg through an exchange of clucking noises; there may be mechanisms of identification between the human mother and the foetus or child that remain to be discovered.

McLaren: This clucking is the equivalent of prenatal uterine influences in our own species. Consider egg transfer from donor (E.T.D.): that is, not the type of egg transfer between husband and wife that Dr Edwards was talking about, but the procedure of taking the egg from a donor woman, B, and then fertilizing it with the sperm from A's husband before placing it in his wife A. This would be analogous to A.I.D. in that the genetic contribution comes from one parent only, but it might raise fewer problems for the marriage relation because the contribution would be more equally shared: the father would contribute the sperm, the mother would provide not the egg but the entire uterine environment throughout pregnancy, which should enhance the mother–child bond. In A.I.D., the mother provides both genetic and uterine contributions and the husband gives nothing prenatally except goodwill.

Mason: On the contrary, the husband of a woman having A.I.D. does have a significant role; he provides for his wife, looks after her during her pregnancy and by the time the baby is born feels that it is his. Presumably he has not abstained from intercourse. His role becomes the same as any other father. We seem to be overlooking the wishes of the couples. We are talking about the moral issues and how we think about it; nobody has mentioned how these couples feel. Do people want A.I.D.? In my opinion there is no doubt that they do; many request it and genuinely want it.

Andrejew: Dr McLaren, what are the arguments against considering the woman A who has the child in her womb as the mother, rather than the donor woman B?

McLaren: This is a question of distinguishing the different types of mother-hood: the genetic (or egg) mother, the uterine (or gestational) mother and the social mother who looks after the baby from birth onwards. From the woman's point of view the uterine, gestational aspect is important.

Andrejew: More important than the genetic mother?

McLaren: I don't think we have any grounds for saying that—I am speaking intuitively—but I definitely think it is important and should not be ignored.

Isaacs: The movement of an infant inside the uterus has a profound psychological effect on the woman. I agree that identity is not only psychological, but since psychology is part of the social environment, psychological factors are important in identity. This does not rule out imprinting, or vice versa.

J. H. Edwards: Canon Dunstan seemed to imply that more information would enable us to act more rationally, particularly if we had registers of genetic identity. Although these registers might be helpful, there is the practical problem of collection of this information.

Male infertility seems to be usually merely functional infertility in that the men appear to be normal in all procedures available for testing, as do their wives (see p. 28). I believe it is unreasonable, and probably impractical, to protect wives from their husbands' sperm while being inseminated with that from another man. I agree that it is extremely irresponsible to mix the semen from donors since this would deny us access to any information, including the capacity of a donor to produce normal children. It is irresponsible to use a donor again if any child with any congenital disease of unknown aetiology, such as spina bifida, resulted. Whether the donor should be informed of this is another matter. Clearly the best test of being able to produce normal children is the production of normal children, and to that extent any person who keeps the records of the donors is responsible for seeing that they are used and not misused. If they are not used they should not be kept.

The danger of a national register is the potential misuse of its information. It could be used locally to assess, first, the fertility of the donor and secondly, whether he can achieve satisfactory results. The inevitable selection of the donor is bound to be unsatisfactory either because the selector chooses what he or she believes to be good characteristics, or because the donor selects himself, with or without money changing hands. The practical uses of a large register escape me in that the ethical questions seem to be almost irrelevant to the sort of information collected. As a guide to the scope for research you could, theoretically, study the proportion of healthy children who pass school exams and live in happy households; but this information is irrelevant, as it is in adoption, because the parents are those whose whole life depends on rearing children, and to that extent one is dealing with an unusual family, for which there are no equivalent control families. So I feel that there is the strongest contraindication to collecting information, except under the highly confidential, localized and restrictive circumstances usual in, for example, records of some psychiatric departments and clinics for venereal disease. I can see neither the genetical nor empirical use for a national register, nor the administrative purpose it would serve; I can see all sorts of potentialities for its misuse.

McLaren: Even though the genetic register which Canon Dunstan proposed might not be very useful, through being erroneous (owing to the possibility that occasionally the supposedly infertile husband fertilizes the egg), our present registry system is itself erroneous in all those cases where the husband is not actually the father of the child. Are there any statistics on how common this is? This is probably more frequent than the cases where a supposedly infertile husband was really the father of an A.I.D. child.

Philipp: We blood-tested some patients in a town in south-east England, and found that 30% of the husbands could not have been the fathers of their children.

Stone: If a man marries a woman he knows to be pregnant by some other person he frequently does not refuse to be registered as the father of her child. Similarly, I understand that in France it is 'the done thing' for a man who marries a woman with an illegitimate child to 'recognize' his paternity of the child although he knows that there is no biological link between them (see p. 71). If the child is illegitimate the woman may not even know the identity of the man, and if she is pressed too hard to give the identity of the putative father, she might tell whatever lie she thinks is most likely to be believed. The Scandinavians ran into a similar difficulty some years ago: they ruled that when an affiliation order was made, not only the man they thought to be the father was ordered to maintain the child, but if there were several men who might have been the father, they all had to contribute. This was found to have a detrimental effect on the child later on, when he was faced with a court finding of his mother's promiscuity at the relevant time. Eventually they decided this was not a good idea. One has to make up one's mind at some point that one has pursued the truth far enough and then let the matter rest.

Stallworthy: I am sure that many doctors would not wish to register the husband as the father of a child if they knew that it had been conceived by A.I.D. They would feel that they were falsifying the records.

Williams: The idea of an impartial duty to keep the records straight seems to me itself rather manipulative.

J. H. Edwards: I was specifically suggesting the danger of a national register for artificial inseminations, not registers as a whole; the Register of Births and Deaths has been, effectively, a genetic register since 1837. This could of course be supplemented by integration and computerization. With advancing knowledge it is surely becoming less and less useful to investigate distant relatives. Genetic diagnosis is becoming increasingly based on biochemistry rather than on heraldry. I doubt whether the limited information which could be acquired from artificial insemination would compensate for the fact that people were being interrogated, and possibly tested, to keep the register accurate. However remote the chance that a conception was within the marriage, in spite of visits to an inseminator, it would not be very helpful psychologically to dismiss it or to rebut it. This would be a consequence of registries, the accuracy of which people start trying to improve as soon as they exist. Accuracy would have little genetic benefit and considerable psychological hazard. My suggestion that registries would not be helpful was irrelevant to the fact that they would probably be more accurate than the data acquired from naturally inseminated families.

Dunstan: I am surprised and slightly disappointed that a scientific body like this has treated so lightheartedly questions of truth and the record of truth. I was trained as a historian and am perhaps more rigorous about this. But the more we discuss the matter, the more it seems to me that accurate and reliable records, both public and private, are essential to any progress, whether social or scientific, in this field.

Kilbrandon: Would historians be seriously disturbed if the records were not accurate in this way?

Williams: A doctor is under no obligation to provide material for future historians. Other things being equal, there clearly are some obligations of this kind; one regrets the dispersal of records, archives and the destruction of material, but people are overimpressed by the idea that they ought to be providing for future historians.

Feilding: While I am greatly attracted by Canon Dunstan's plea for a privileged record of biological parentage (in addition to the open and normal register of births), I am compelled to wonder, with Professor J. H. Edwards, what use it would be. The difficulty, as I now see it, is compounded by the uncertainties concerning the alleged facts of parentage. Do the standards now upheld in medical practice and in the present state of our knowledge demand that such facts should be routinely discovered and recorded for all? Could the record, however threatening to privacy on the one hand and however useful for the study of trends on the other, be relied on in medical practice in dealing with a specific individual? I do not intend these questions to be rhetorical as this would presume to more knowledge of the data than I possess.

Graham: As I understand it, the general practice in the U.K. now is that the A.I.D. child is not told about his origins. Professor Fried suggested that in the United States this was becoming a problem in various matrimonial and other related cases, where eventually the child came to know because of the judicial proceedings. Even if the secret of his origins is kept from the child for as long as possible, most likely the child will discover it in adolescence, during the sort of arguments that most healthy adolescents have with their parents, when they are concerned about themselves and their independence. I am concerned about children learning about their genetic origin at that particular time, when their identity is in a state of greater confusion than at practically any other time of their lives. At the moment, when the procedure is regarded as of doubtful ethical status, there may be special problems in telling the children, but I believe this is a strong argument in favour of clarifying the status of the procedure.

Academically, one can distinguish biological, genetic and social parentage; this is no problem. As far as the affected individual's perception of himself is concerned, the situation may be much more confused. It is all very well to say that the donor (that is, the genetic father) must not be involved but perhaps some donors are, despite themselves, troubled by thoughts of children they may have fathered.

Mason: Whether the couples tell their children is to a large extent up to the couples themselves. Of those women Mr Philipp referred to (p. 63), how many told either the child or her husband? I imagine very few. A similar argument applies to A.I.D. Dr Graham, have you ever had an A.I.D. child under your care? Have you ever seen psychological problems in them?

Graham: The short answer is 'not knowingly'. There are things that psychiatrists never get to know, believe it or not!

Mason: By now many A.I.D. babies have grown up, married and had children. If people in your position have never come across a child who has had psychological problems attributed to his A.I.D. identity, maybe we are worrying about things that are rare. I am sure that problems will arise, but not with every A.I.D. baby.

Graham: If we *never* encounter problems in A.I.D. children this would strongly suggest that the whole system was operating on denial because one would expect to find disturbance in 6–7% of children in the general population. The fact that I have not seen disturbed children born by A.I.D. indicates that, if the practice is as prevalent as you have suggested, there are problems of denial. By analogy, one is rarely told at a first interview (or even after many subsequent interviews) that children are the products of extramarital affairs. All the same, one knows that this is not an uncommon situation (p. 63).

Kilbrandon: Mr Philipp, surely the figure of 30% must be a minimum? What you established was that 30% could not be the children of their mothers' husbands, not that 70% of them were?

Philipp: Yes, it is a minimum. We were screening some female patients by testing their husbands for their blood groups, because we were interested in antibody formation in correlation with the ABO groups as well as the rhesus groups. From our results we suddenly realized that 30% of the children could not have been fathered by the men whose blood groups we had analysed.

Stallworthy: What was the extent of that group?

Philipp: Not large—between 200 and 300 women—but large enough to give us a great shock.

J. H. Edwards: There are various biases due to the social conditions which determine delivery in hospital rather than at home: these include primiparity, especially when conception precedes marriage. Analysis of some blood group data, making allowance for the fact that one could not detect all the illegitimacies, showed that in the 1950s in the West Isleworth area about 50% of premarital conceptions were not fathered by the apparent father.[1] As the apparent fathers were questioned while visiting their wives immediately after the birth, most of them obviously thought they were the father. I think the group Mr Philipp referred to is also highly biased. In spite of much talk about artificial insemination by donor and all the difficulties with genetics and so on, natural insemination by donor is practised on quite a substantial scale on an amateur basis. There is no doubt that many rhesus-sensitized women do manage to overcome their difficulties, apparently without disrupting their marriages.

Williams: Dr Graham's distinction of roles is not going to solve the problems of parents and donors now. But as his remarks about fantasy illustrated (p. 34), certain sorts of confusion of identity are essential to the process of growing up —a number of ordinary legitimate children fantasize that they are adopted or illegitimate. No doubt A.I.D. will become part of that fantasy, if it has not already done so. I do not want to deny that for a moment. I was relating my remarks more to Professor Fried's suggestion that we should think about the nature of the system if we had a different general institutional pattern. What is the obstacle to dissociating the roles of genetic father and social father in general?

Stallworthy: We should remember that we are living in times when attitudes are changing very quickly, so much so that in some of the civilized societies (privileged countries) the sense of genetic responsibility from a social point of view is such that society is willing to destroy at least half its pregnancies by abortion. It is easy in a group like this to forget that this is the prevalent climate. We should take this into account when considering some of the pronouncements which have been made.

Bevis: How can any society that accepts termination of pregnancy quibble about the giving of life to a foetus? We are not creating life. If we can kill the foetus— and this seems to be expected and accepted—why can we not 'put it together'?

Perutz: If you kill a foetus nothing happens, there will be no child, but if you 'put together' a child, you might produce an unhappy individual. The responsibility is of a different kind.

Bevis: But there can also be great changes in the mother and often in the father.

Williams: The killing of a foetus does not introduce a new social role: there is that difference. I agree that the attitude to abortion shows that much that is said about genetic responsibility is rubbish. Many facts about society bear this out—the 30% of the children somewhere in south-east England for one (p. 63)! But the practice of abortion does not introduce the two different social roles of the genetic father and the social father.

McLaren: Canon Dunstan pointed out that it was the atmosphere of social and moral disapproval surrounding A.I.D. at present that largely prevented us from making a moral assessment of many of these issues. Dr Graham was making basically the same point by implying that such an atmosphere prevents the psychological assessment of A.I.D. children, since he does not know which of his patients, if any, were conceived through A.I.D. Probably A.I.D. children should be told their origins, like adopted children, as early as possible, but in the present atmosphere it is neither desirable nor possible. This is not because of any doubts about the legality of A.I.D., but rather because of the present status of illegitimacy of A.I.D. children.

Kilbrandon: More than once it has been implied that the procedure of A.I.D. is illegal. I know of no law which prohibits it.

Graham: But the legal status of those who are born in this way lacks clarification.

Kilbrandon: It seems that some practitioners are dubious about carrying out the procedure because they are afraid it was illegal. Nobody has yet suggested any law against it.

References

[1] EDWARDS, J. H. (1957) A critical examination of the reputed primary influence of ABO phenotype on fertility and sex ratio. *British Journal of Preventive and Social Medicine* **11**, 79–89

[2] HANACK, Professor (1972) German Gynaecological Congress, Wiesbaden, summarized by W. Cyran (1973), *Frankfurter Allgemeine*, 3rd January

[3] HESS, E. H. (1972) 'Imprinting' in a natural laboratory. *Scientific American* **227**, 24–31

[4] MITTLER, P. (1971) *The Study of Twins*, Penguin Books, Harmondsworth, Middlesex

[5] TIEVARI, P. (1966) On intrapair differences in male twins. *Acta Psychiatrica Scandinavica (Supplementum)* **188**, 42

[6] TITMUSS, R. M. (1971) *The Gift Relationship: from human blood to social policy*, Allen & Unwin, London

[7] U.K. Law Commission (1973) *Injuries to Unborn Children*, Published Working Paper no. 47

[8] ZAZZO, R. (1960) *Les Jumeaux: le Couple et la Personne*, Presses Universitaires de France, Paris

English law in relation to A.I.D. and embryo transfer

OLIVE M. STONE

A.I.D.

(a) Consents

The woman recipient of A.I.D. must, of course, consent to the treatment, and for purposes of evidence such consents should be in writing. After 1969, it seems that any woman over the age of 16 can validly consent.[1]

There is no legal requirement that if the woman is married her husband should consent. If he does not do so, it is clear that the treatment does not amount to adultery by the wife.[2] Adultery involves sexual intercourse between two persons, at least one of whom is married, but who are not married to each other. Sexual intercourse for this purpose must involve some penetration, however slight, of the female by the male organ.[3] It seems probable, however, that if a wife underwent such treatment without her husband's consent and he objected, considered that the marriage had broken down irretrievably and petitioned for

---

[1] The Family Law Reform Act 1969, s.8 reads: 'The consent of a minor who has attained the age of sixteen years to any surgical, medical or dental treatment which, in the absence of consent, would constitute a trespass to his person, shall be as effective as it would be if he were of full age; and where a minor has by virtue of this section given an effective consent to any treatment it shall not be necessary to obtain any consent for it from his parent or guardian'.

[2] The Scottish Court of Session so held in *Maclennan* v. *Maclennan* [1958] *Scots Law Times* 12, and the decision is generally accepted as good law in England also. In the United States, the Illinois Court held in *Doornbos* v. *Doornbos* (1956), 12 Ill. App. 2d 473, 139 N.E.2d in a divorce case, that a child born as the result of A.I.D. was not a legitimate child and that the use of A.I.D. constituted adultery. An appeal was dismissed. In the unreported case of *Hock* v. *Hock* (1945) an Illinois court held that artificial insemination did not establish adultery as ground for divorce. There was a similar decision in Ontario in 1921: *Oxford* v. *Oxford* (1921) 58 *Dominion Law Reports* 251.

[3] *Dennis* v. *Dennis* [1955] *P.* 153.

divorce, it might be held that she had behaved in such a way that he could not reasonably be expected to live with her[4] and his petition be granted.

(b) The sperm used

Medical practice appears to favour the purchase of sperm from donors whose identity is known only to the medical practitioner, who is satisfied of the donor's physical health. The literature suggests that the donor may deliver the sperm to the medical practitioner, presumably with an undertaking as to its origin. If it should transpire that the child born has traits not anticipated by the practitioner or desired by the mother (e.g. if the child is of greatly different racial origin or is born with a disease such as syphilis inherited and not from the mother, or if the sperm used could not have emanated from the reputed donor) the mother might be able to sustain an action for damages for negligence or misrepresentation against the medical practitioner. There is also the possibility of an action for damages by the child against the medical practitioner for birth with some physical defect. This could not be barred by any consent given by the mother or any other person. Actions against the suppliers of thalidomide by those born with physical defects as a result of the use of the drug by the mother during pregnancy are still pending in the courts.[5]

(c) Registration of birth

The Births and Deaths Registration Acts[6] require the birth of the child to be registered by entering in a register 'such particulars as may be prescribed'. These

---

[4] Under the Divorce Reform Act 1969, s.2(1)(b). Both the Royal Commission on Human Artificial Insemination, in Cmd.9678 para.90, and the Departmental Committee on the same subject in Cmnd.1105 paras.114–117, recommended that artificial insemination of the wife without the husband's consent should be a ground for divorce. The radical amendment of the grounds for divorce operative after 1970 have made such a specific provision unnecessary.

[5] In *Distillers Co. (Biochemicals) Ltd.* v. *Thompson* [1971] *A.C.* 458, the Privy Council advised that a child born with defects in New South Wales had a cause of action against the English company that had sold to an Australian company the Distaval (containing thalidomide) bought by the plaintiff's mother in Australia. In Re *Taylor's Application* [1972] *Q.B.* 369 the Court of Appeal had to consider the proposed settlement by the Distillers Co. of about £3 250 000 on trustees to be used in their discretion for the children concerned. The Court of Appeal held that those parents who assented to the arrangements proposed were not entitled to have the minority of dissenting parents replaced by the Official Solicitor as next friend of their children. On 20th October 1972 the Attorney General obtained an injunction to stop the intended publication in *The Sunday Times* of articles about thalidomide investigations. Subsequent discussions in Parliament led to government provision of funds for handicapped children on 29th November 1972.

[6] The principal Act now operative is the Births and Deaths Registration Act 1953, but sections

include the name and status of the mother and that of the father if known. Lord Kilbrandon has suggested that the term 'father or accepting husband' might be substituted for 'father'.

A child born to a married woman as a result of A.I.D. is the child not of the wife and the husband but of the wife and a man whose identity is unknown to all but the medical practitioner. The child should therefore at present be registered as of illegitimate birth, father unknown. The mother and her husband should then apply to adopt the child. The mother cannot give her consent to any adoption until the child is six weeks old[7] and, before an adoption order can be made, the child must have been in the continuous care and possession of the proposed adopters for at least three months, not including any period before the child was six weeks old.[8] No adoption proceedings can therefore be taken until at least four and a half months after the child's birth.

These provisions are likely to prove frustrating to both husband and wife, and the uncertainty that must remain until the adoption order has been finally made will probably involve considerable strain on both of them.[9] The child must also be told that he is adopted, since he will obtain only a short form of birth certificate and must have a court order before he can obtain a copy of his original birth record. How much more he should be told will be a matter for consideration.

It is widely accepted that some degree of falsification of birth registers now takes place. If a man marries a woman whom he knows to be pregnant by some other person he will not infrequently declare himself to be the father of the child when born.[10] This prevents the official notification of matters thought to concern only the immediate parties, and helps to stop gossip. Probably no great harm ensues, as the true facts are known at least to the mother and probably to

---

of the Acts of 1836, 1837, 1856, 1858, 1874 and 1926 are still in operation, in addition to the Census Act 1920, and the Population (Statistics) Act 1938. The penalties generally provided under the Acts and under the Non-Parochial Registers Act 1840 are not specific.

[7] Adoption Act 1958, s.6(2)

[8] Adoption Act 1958, s.3(1)

[9] In Cmnd.5107 published 4th October 1972, the Stockdale Departmental Committee on the Adoption of Children has now resiled from its earlier recommendation that a natural parent should never be permitted to adopt his or her child, and now recommends (No. 20) that 'where a relative (including a step-parent applying jointly with his spouse) applies to adopt a child, the law should require the court first to consider whether guardianship would be more appropriate in all the circumstances of the case, first consideration being given to the long-term welfare of the child'.

[10] In a recent private discussion between Belgian, French and English lawyers, nobody was prepared to recommend pursuing such pious perjury with all the legal penalties provided. For these, as for other offences, the police have considerable discretionary powers. I understand that in France, when a man marries the mother of an illegitimate child, it is considered 'the done thing' for him to 'recognize' paternity of the child, even though he has no biological connection with it.

her husband, and could be disclosed if, for example, marriage within the prohibited degrees appeared likely. The probability of harm decreases once the
child marries, and generally with the passage of time. But with the child born of
A.I.D. the position is different, since no one except the medical practitioner
knows the identity of the father. If a false declaration is made serious consequences might result, quite apart from the penalties that might be incurred.[11]

The above suggests that (i) the medical practitioner should make some record
of the identity of the donor to be kept for (say) 50 years, with special provisions about who should have access to the record and in what circumstances,
and (ii) new legal provisions may be desirable, either to amend the description
of the child's male parent, or to enable the parties, at the time of the treatment,
to make an application to adopt jointly any child resulting from it and to adopt
the child while *en ventre sa mère*, contingent on its being born alive. Then at birth
the child will be the legally adopted child of the husband and wife, and will not
only become so at some later time if an application then made is successful.
Some might prefer a provision that the child born of A.I.D. with the husband's
consent should be considered the legitimate child of the mother and her husband
and so registered.

(d) Legality of A.I.D. in the United States

In the United States, the States of California, Georgia and Oklahoma have
all provided by statute that the practice of A.I.D. is legal and that the children
born of the treatment are the legitimate children of the wife and her husband,
provided the latter has given his written consent. Similar legislation has been
rejected in Indiana, Minnesota, New York, Virginia and Wisconsin. Ohio rejected a Bill which would have rendered A.I.D. a criminal offence by both the
woman and her physician. However, in the State of New York, it was held in
Strnad v. *Strnad*[12] that, where a child had been born of A.I.D. to which the
husband had given his written consent, the child was not illegitimate, but was in
the position of an adopted child or a child born out of wedlock and legitimated

---

[11] The most convenient and frequently used are those under the Perjury Act 1911, s.4, which
provides that if anyone '(1)(a) wilfully gives to a registrar any false information concerning any
birth or death, or (b) wilfully makes any false certificate or declaration under or for the purposes
of any Act relating to the registration of births or deaths, or ... (d) makes any false statement with
intent to have the same inserted in any register of births or deaths; he is guilty of a misdemeanour,
liable (i) on conviction on indictment to imprisonment for a term not exceeding seven years or a
fine or both, and (ii) on summary conviction to a penalty not exceeding one hundred pounds'.
No prosecution on indictment may be begun more than three years after commission of the
offence.
[12] (1948) 190 Misc. 786, 78 N.Y. S.2d 390

by the marriage of his parents. In *People* v. *Sorrenson*[31] a Californian Court held that, where a child had been born of A.I.D. to which the husband had given his written consent, the husband was criminally liable for failure to support the child, of which he was the father within the meaning of the criminal code.

(e) *Insurance*

For life insurance purposes, presumably the disclosure of the known facts and a catalogue of those unknown would be needed before the child or anyone else could effect insurance on his life. The medical adviser in possession of the facts would presumably consider it his duty to reveal the facts he knew to the insurance company at the request of the adoptive parents or the child.

EMBRYO TRANSFER

(a) As distinct from A.I.D., on which the first reported decision appears to be that of the court of Bordeaux in 1883, embryo transfer is so far only the subject of animal experiments. I understand that the work contemplated by Drs Edwards and Steptoe will be restricted to facilitating the birth of children genealogically descended from married couples, where the wife suffers from some maternal disability, such as tubal occlusion. In this procedure an unfertilized human embryo would be removed by laparoscopy, fertilized with the husband's sperm and grown on *in vitro* until the stage at which the embryo would normally enter the uterus. The embryo would then be surgically implanted in the mother's uterus, and normal gestation and birth would follow.

Such a procedure would give rise to no legal problems apart from the possibility of teratology, or induced foetal deformities, for which heavy damages might be recoverable.

Lord Kilbrandon has compared such a procedure to facilitating birth by Caesarian section. If successful it will result in the birth to the woman of a child of whom her husband is the biological father. Biological and legal relationship will coincide, as for the vast majority of births. Since England has no statutory definition of a legitimate or an illegitimate child, drafting difficulties are unlikely to arise.[14] Biological father and mother will both be correctly registered as the parents of the child.

---

[13] (1968) 60 Cal. Rptr. 495, 437 P.2d 495

[14] They may arise in other jurisdictions. For example, New York City's Criminal Courts Act declares illegitimate the children of a married woman 'begotten at a time when the husband is impotent' [see Ploscowe, M. (1948) Your test-tube baby may be illegitimate. *Lawyers Guild Review* **8**, 496].

Problems might arise if at some later time the husband wished to contend that by some chance, mistake, or deception he was not in fact the biological father of the the child born. The presumption of law that a husband is the father of his wife's child remains, but after 1969,[15] although the burden will be on the husband to show that he was not the father, this will be less difficult than it was before 1970. The medical adviser might be called upon to show what precautions were taken to ensure that only the husband's sperm was used.

(b) Blood tests

These may show that a particular man or woman could not be the father or mother of a particular child or, on the other hand, that he could be and that only a very small proportion of the general population could have filled such a role because of the presence of rare characteristics.[16] If a man who doubts the paternity of his child can obtain his wife's agreement to the administration of blood tests to herself and, should he not have custody of the child, to the child as well, no legal problems arise. If agreement cannot be obtained, since 1st March 1972 the court may direct that blood tests be administered.[17]

Anybody who has attained the age of 16 may consent to blood tests on himself.[18] The court cannot compel an unwilling person to take blood tests but if it gives a direction for blood tests to be taken and 'any person fails to take any step required of him for the purpose of giving effect to the direction, the court may draw such inferences, if any, from that fact as appear proper in the circumstance',[19] and need not apply the presumption of legitimacy.[20]

---

[15]   Family Law Reform Act 1969, s.26: 'Any presumption of law as to the legitimacy or illegitimacy of any person may in any civil proceedings be rebutted by evidence which shows that it is more probable than not that that person is illegitimate or legitimate, as the case may be, and it shall not be necessary to prove that fact beyond reasonable doubt in order to rebut the presumption.'

[16]   The information given in Appendix B to Law Com. No. 16: *Blood Tests and the Proof of Paternity in Civil Proceedings*, published 1968, is already somewhat out of date.

[17]   Family Law Reform Act 1969, s.20: 'In any civil proceedings in which the paternity of any person falls to be determined by the court hearing the proceedings the court may, on an application by any party to the proceedings, give a direction for the use of blood tests to ascertain whether such tests show that a party to the proceedings is or is not thereby excluded from being the father of that person and for the taking, within a period to be specified in the direction, of blood samples from that person, the mother of the person and any party alleged to be the father of that person or from any, or any two, of those persons'.

[18]   Family Law Reform Act 1969, s.21(2)

[19]   Family Law Reform Act 1969, s.23

[20]   Family Law Reform Act 1969, s.23(2)

(c) Consents and possible claims or penalties

As the treatment involves surgery, it is attended by greater risks of injury. The written consent of both parents would be essential, but they could not bind the child. There would presumably be no difficulty in showing that all stages of the treatment were for the patient's benefit and lawfully justified.[21] Removal of an unfertilized embryo would not appear to amount to abortion. Removal of a fertilized embryo, on the other hand, would be illegal unless justified on grounds of necessity under the *Bourne*[22] doctrine or falling within the terms of the Abortion Act 1967.

(d) If the range of possible treatment were later to be extended to removal of an embryo from one woman and insertion after fertilization in the uterus of another woman, further questions might arise. It would be necessary to show that removal of the embryo was for the benefit of the woman from whom it was removed, as well as for the benefit of the recipient woman. The question of maternal rights as between the ovum mother and the uterine mother might present difficulty, but it is not thought that maternal rights are likely to inhere in the supplier of an unfertilized embryo. If partial parental rights were involved, a court order would be needed to terminate them, since they cannot be effectively renounced.[23]

As the law now stands, only when, as the result of an application to it, the court has made an adoption order, is the situation reached that 'all rights, duties, obligations and liabilities of the parents ... of the infant, in relation to the future custody, maintenance and education of the infant, including all rights to appoint a guardian and ... to consent or give notice of dissent to marriage, shall be extinguished, and all such rights, duties, obligations and liabilities shall vest in and be exercisable by and enforceable against the adopter as if the infant were a child born to the adopter in lawful wedlock'.[24]

(e) Registration of birth

If the embryo and the sperm used are those of the uterine mother and her

---

[21] See Dworkin, G. (1970) *The Law Relating to Organ Transplantation in England*, 33 *Modern Law Review* 353. This article does not specifically consider embryo transplants.
[22] *Rex* v. *Bourne* [1939] 1 *K.B.* 687
[23] In *Re F* [1957] 1 *All E.L.R.* 819, the father of a legitimate child, believing the mother to be incurably of unsound mind, renounced all parental rights to the child by deed. No adoption order having been made, the parents were able to recover the child when the mother recovered (as she rapidly did).
[24] Adoption Act 1958, s.13

husband, no problems arise. If a fertilized embryo had been transferred from another woman, the father's identity might be unknown, as would be that of the embryo mother. The uterine mother would be identifiable in all cases. If in the future there is a real possibility of division of the maternal role, legislation would be desirable to clarify whether the uterine mother is entitled to be registered as the child's mother and if so, whether any indication should be given of her special capacity.

SELECT BIBLIOGRAPHY

On artificial insemination

PLOSCOWE, M., FOSTER, H. H., JR. & FREED, D. J. (1972) (*Family Law, Cases and Materials*, 2nd edn., Little, Brown, Boston & Toronto) list the considerable American and British literature on the subject, of which the following is a small selection:
BARTHOLOMEW, G. W. (1958) Legal implications of artificial insemination, 21 *Modern Law Review* 236
HARGROVE, B. (1958) Artificial insemination by donor, 25 *Solicitor* 165
KELLY, G. (1956) Artificial insemination: a symposium, 33 *University of Detroit Law Journal* 135
O'RAHILLY, R. (1957) Artificial insemination: a symposium, 34 *University of Detroit Law Journal* 383
POLLARD, R. S. W. (1961) Report of the department committee on human artificial insemination, 24 *Modern Law Review* 158
PUXTON, M. (1960) Legitimacy and artificial insemination, 104 *Solicitors' Journal* 575

On organ transplants generally

DWORKIN, G. (1970) The law relating to organ transplantation in England, 33 *Modern Law Review* 353, and literature there cited n. 2
KILBRANDON, BARON (1966) in *Ethics in Medical Progress (Ciba Foundation Symposium)*, Churchill, London

Legal aspects of artificial insemination and embryo transfer in French domestic law and private international law

MARIEL REVILLARD

Far from remaining insensitive to the repercussions of scientific discoveries, civil law has evolved under the influence of progress in biology. This is to be expected if we admit, as we do in all western democracies, that the object of civil law is not to impose strict rules based on religious, political or racial assumptions but to try to derive empirically a set of standards to ensure the protection of people in both their individual lives and their social relations. Civil law must be constantly revised to adapt to the consequences of technological progress.[25] The biologist who handles life for the benefit of mankind must do so without legal constraint. But one day the scientist will need lawyers to help him reconcile the applications of his discovery with respect for the individual. Methods of intensive care which allow organisms to be maintained artificially have already compelled the traditional criteria of death to be reconsidered and the concept of cerebral death to be defined. This medico-legal work was no mere intellectual exercise but was necessary to allow the removal of organs for transplantation from a donor after his cerebral death.[30] A few years after having had to reconsider their biologically naive conception of death, lawyers now have to question their traditional criteria of affiliation and define the moment at which a fertilized egg can be considered as an individual.

Until now, the French lawyer has prudently ignored the definition of the beginning of an individual's life. Roman Catholic teaching considers that life begins at fertilization; others fix the time at implantation. Administrative rules and French jurisprudence require the registration of embryos more than 180 days old, and recommend the declaration of embryos after the sixth week of gestation according to a regulation dating back to 1868.[17] Article 317 of the Penal Code, which defines and sanctions abortion, mentions 'the premature expulsion of the foetus' or more generally 'the interruption of pregnancy' without stating the stage of embryonic development after which this action can be considered as criminal. The concern of jurisprudence is more with the intention of interrupting pregnancy than with the biological criterion of the size of the embryo. If the lawyers have not deemed it necessary to use precise biological data in this field, it would not be surprising if they were unable to establish a satisfactory code for artificial insemination and embryo implantation.

The study of this problem in French law is now of great interest on account of the reform of the law of affiliation brought in by the Decree of 3rd January 1972. This Decree did not touch on the problem of artificial insemination. The legislators do not seem to have wanted to accept the full consequences of a purely genetic analysis of affiliation. The technique of artificial insemination entails the revision of one of the postulates on which the law of affiliation in the French Civil Code rests: it is no longer true to say that a birth is necessarily the result of the father and mother coming together physically.[34] Embryo transfer brings into question the notion of kinship and maternal affiliation which, until now, had been considered as incontestable on the principle *mater semper certa est.*

The basis of any legal analysis of affiliation is the concept that each individual is the product of both his genetic patrimony and his environment. The legal aspects of this dualism are well illustrated by adoption. In the absence of any hereditary link between the adopter and adopted, the reform of the law of adoption (Decree, 11th July 1966) gave the adopted child the same rights as a legitimate child within the limits of *adoption plénière* (Civil Code, Art. 358 and ref. 24). The situation in which the adopted child is no longer a stranger to his adopting parents with whom he has no genetic link will be one of the bases of our reasoning, especially in the case of a child genetically issued from only one of the parents. Where legitimate affiliation is concerned, the presumption *pater is est* can cover many situations that are unacceptable to genetics and, on the whole, French legislators have tried to consolidate the idea of the family, concerning themselves fundamentally more with appearances than biological truth.

Before we try to justify or limit the application of artificial insemination and embryo transfer, we must ascertain their object. Apart from pure research, these techniques have essentially one therapeutic purpose: the treatment of sterility. But what is sterility? Legally, sterility can be considered within the limits of the family and the marriage institution. In French positive law, the impossibility of procreation or the desire not to have children is neither an obstacle to marriage nor a cause for invalidity of marriage or for divorce. Only the concealment of such a condition or the refusal to submit to medical treatment is regarded as a serious injury which, in some cases, may form grounds for a divorce.[1]

Medically, is sterility a physical handicap or an illness? The physician who treats an illness, especially when the risks in treatment or inherent in the disease could lead to a fatal outcome, is not under any duty or contract to produce results, but is obliged to show prudence and diligence; that is, his duty lies in the means. In this context, he is able to run some risks in taking advantage of the latest therapeutic discoveries. Any therapy, even the most widely used, always entails a risk. The physician must evaluate the risk of the treatment against the consequences of the illness itself.[31] Conversely, in plastic surgery, for example, which is generally used for physical disabilities that handicap patients without endangering their lives, the doctor is bound by law to achieve satisfactory results.

What, then, is the legal position of the treatment of sterility? Procreation is a legitimate aspiration for every individual. In our opinion sterility should be considered as a physical disability and can be regarded as an illness only when it causes psychiatric disturbances. Again the risks of treatment must be weighed against those of sterility itself. It is therefore medical criteria and not the application of a technique that help to define the limits of acceptable procedures. Although technically we are able to make an absolute choice, we are still bound by the medical objective when this technique is used. Just as the essential condition for adoption in French law is the absence of any legitimate descendant, so the use of artificial insemination and embryo transfer should be permissible only in the absence of any descendant and when procreation is impossible for medical reasons.

Of course, it is not unlikely that these stipulations will have to be reconsidered in the future. Nobody would now contest that complete freedom in the choice of a husband or wife constitutes one of the essential rights of the individual, even though in some countries the wife is bought and therefore finds herself compelled to take a certain husband. This makes us realize the relativity of our legal concepts in connection with socio-psychological and historical data. We can no longer exclude the possibility that in a few decades, when our western civilization has reached the climax of its matriarchal period, the wife will consider the free choice of her descendants independently of her husband, through the use of sperm banks, as one of her essential rights. This right can be considered to be acquired in practice in French law, in that at present a married woman can recognize an illegitimate child while the state of marriage exists (Civil Code, Art. 313–1), even if the obligation of faithfulness subsists and is penalized in criminal law (adultery) and civil law (divorce).

Lawyers must learn to distrust the sensationalism and public outcry based on insufficient knowledge about new techniques and treatments. After Sir Peter Medawar's work on tissue grafts it seemed likely that the very definition of a human being was going to be questioned again; some people imagined that the concept of an individual would be destroyed by grafting brain, just as others naively believed that the soul was changed through blood transfusion. The transplantation of organs has saved many human lives and it has not been necessary to draft laws to limit brain grafts to pure research to further our understanding of some neurological diseases. This, I think, well illustrates the limits of the medical applications within which we should work.

ARTIFICIAL INSEMINATION

The legal aspects of artificial insemination depend on the kind of intervention, that is on whether the sperm comes from the husband (A.I.H.) or a donor A.I.D.). Medically, insemination of the wife with the husband's semen cannot be considered as artificial insemination but rather as an aid to natural insemination. Accurate statistics on A.I.H. are not available, but A.I.D. is practised on about 1000 couples annually in France. The French Civil Code ignores artificial insemination, and other countries have no code either. However, in Denmark and Scandinavia, an advice on insemination has existed since 1948 but it has never been enacted.[19]

A judgement on artificial insemination exists in French jurisprudence (Bordeaux Civil Court, 27th August 1883; the suit has been entered into as a claim for medical fees). The procedure is alluded to in only two other proceedings, one for divorce (Lyon, 28th May 1956, ref. 4), the other for disavowal (Paris, 10th February 1956, S. 1956. 20). In the absence of other precedents, we must use legal principles to evaluate the medical responsibility in artificial insemination and the effects of artificial insemination on the law of affiliation.

Medical responsibility and artificial insemination

Artificial insemination can be considered as a medical contract and therefore can be dealt with in criminal and civil law.

Criminal aspects. At present no law forbids artificial insemination or its practice in France. However, the practitioner runs the risk of being an accessory to acts amounting to infringement of criminal law, such as indecent behaviour, adultery or simply constraint (Penal Code, Art. 311).[18]

Is insemination of a woman by force rape? Certainly not: sexual conjunction, which is the material element of rape, is absent. Such action is not rape but indecent behaviour with constraint or voluntary constraint with malice aforethought.[36]

Does artificial insemination of a consenting married woman without her husband's knowledge or consent constitute adultery? Would the doctor be an accessory?[10, 27] Suppose a married woman has herself inseminated without her husband's knowledge, in the hope that she will bear an exceptionally gifted child. In France, as in Italy and West Germany, criminal law does not define adultery but merely punishes it. The jurisprudential premise of the conjunction of the woman and her lover thus excludes the possibility of the doctor or the sperm donor being an accessory. But such clandestine insemination certainly constitutes serious injury to the husband and forms grounds for a divorce suit.

The doctor can also be criminally responsible through complicity with the husband: should a doctor conspire with a sterile husband, who wants to hide his physical disability from his wife, to substitute semen from a donor for that of the husband, the doctor would be criminally responsible if this was revealed (and proved!). If the doctor inseminated the wife by force, even with the husband's sperm, he would have committed the offence of constraint to which the husband would be an accessory. Conversely, the use of a husband's semen on a woman other than his wife cannot be claimed as adultery by his wife.

These examples may appear to be fanciful ideas of lawyers. However, the contract between the practitioner, the donor and the sterile couple embodies certain obligations characteristic of any medical contract.

Civil aspects. The need for artificial insemination is never urgent and the procedure should remain a method of treatment for childless couples. Let us now consider the analogy with adoption.[6]

Artificial insemination raises a problem of legal capacity and concerns people who are of age and qualified to enter into a contract. The impossibility of procreation must be established as being due to sterility. Only when the sterility has been recognized as incurable is medical intervention possible. The wish for a child must be normal and lasting. The practitioner must judge the future parents suitable to educate and keep the child; obviously, the child should enter a home where both father and mother want him. In France, most physicians are opposed to the insemination of an unmarried woman who lives alone. However, in view of the sociological evolution of the family and the rights granted to the natural child by the recent reform of the law of affiliation, we see no reason to forbid the insemination of a young unmarried woman with her lover's sperm if the lover is determined to acknowledge the resulting child. That child, thus wanted, would be born into a natural family. Some *concubinages* are as stable as a marriage consecrated by the Registrar. If insemination is reserved for married couples, the physician would have to check the identities of interested parties and ask to see the marriage licence (or equivalent).[18]

The written consent of husband and wife places the responsibility with the sterile couple but does not discharge the practitioner of his responsibility, since a clause of non-responsibility is not valid in these circumstances. It should be noted that the consent given by the father-to-be is not equivalent to renunciation in disavowal proceedings.[35]

It is the practitioner's duty to choose a donor who is mentally and physically sound and who has procreated only healthy children.[6, 8, 9] The practitioner is bound to professional secrecy about the identity of the donor and clearly must refuse members of the husband's family as donors. A child should not know the circumstances of his conception, and the husband and wife are advised to keep the insemination a secret from both their families. The husband and wife should be left free to inform the child at their discretion that he is the descendant of only one of them.

Is the practitioner of artificial insemination obliged to guarantee the results of his treatment or is he only bound by a duty of care? If the procedure fails, would the physician be responsible? Certainly not. The physician is only obliged to prescribe the best possible treatment and to observe the usual conditions of prudence and diligence proper to any medical contract and he is not compelled to ensure the result, that is to say, fertilization. Of course, the doctor is responsible if the operation is performed negligently, thereby causing either failure or infection, or if a geneticist can establish proof of other regrettable consequences, such as negligence allowing the transmission of a hereditary disease.[5]

Even with A.I.H., the doctor's responsibility does not go beyond the intervention itself. Thus, a couple cannot reproach the doctor for a difficult pregnancy or the birth of an abnormal child. But what is the doctor's responsibility in A.I.D., if a child is born with hereditary taints attributable to the donor selected by the practitioner? We say 'attributable': the proof would be intrinsically impossible to make, the donor being anonymous.

The real difficulty for the practitioner lies in deciding whether treatment is indicated and in preserving professional secrecy, which is of paramount importance (see below).

Artificial insemination and affiliation

Our reflections on illegitimate affiliation are theoretical, since artificial fertilization, in principle, concerns married people. If the inseminated woman is unmarried, her child will be illegitimate. If the donor is the woman's lover, paternity can be proved by the normal methods of affiliation or action for affiliation. If the donor is unknown—as, for example, if a girl wanted to have a child without having any relations with a man—there is no question of affiliation to a father; any such action would meet with the professional secrecy of the practitioner, who would preserve the anonymity of the donor. The donor therefore can have no obligation of maintenance towards the child and its mother.

Let us now consider legitimate affiliation. No difficulties should arise in A.I.H. since the husband and wife agree to the insemination. But, suppose that a husband denies paternity of a child on account of the physical separation of the couple (non-access) at the relevant time, while the wife claims the proof of artificial insemination from his own seed.[13] Since 1st August 1972 the husband can attempt to deny paternity by every means at his disposal (Code Civil, Art. 340). Non-access by the husband is no longer in itself a ground for denial since the husband can have his wife inseminated while she is separated from him, with her agreement. Before this reform, artificial insemination was considered to be included in the legal notion of cohabitation. Apparently, the magistrate will refuse denial of paternity whenever the child is born from the husband's seed (cf. ref. 11). Under such conditions, the development of sperm banks and insemination of the woman in the absence of the donor could set more problems in the future.

Does this mean that legitimate children could be conceived *post mortem*? The Civil Code (Arts. 312 and 315) put an end to such futuristic hypotheses. Although the father of a child born during wedlock is presumed to be the husband, the presumption of paternity is not applicable to a child born more than 300 days after the husband's death or disappearance and an action for affiliation would not be allowed (Code Civil, Art. 340). Thus the use of sperm from a sperm bank for A.I.H. must be limited to medical procedures, the performance of which is subject to the agreement of the two living parents capable of bringing up a child together.

A.I.D. is more complex. French legal doctrine has long tried to reconcile A.I.D. with a theory of denied paternity. Thus a child born to a married woman after artificial insemination by a donor who is not her husband cannot be described from the biological point of view by any other term than adulterine.[7] A.I.D. leads to forgery in the child's birth certificate, but the forgery is covered by the legal presumption of the husband's paternity. A husband regretting his apparent paternity could easily substantiate the denial of paternity. The commission for reform of the Civil Code in 1950[38] was occupied with making such denial impossible.

The commission decided that a legal document was not suitable and the project was abandoned, to the satisfaction of many lawyers who had independently concluded that medical secrecy was sufficient guarantee.[18, 23, 28] Since the Decree of 3rd January 1972, any evidence is admissible to rebut the presumption of paternity (Civil Code, Art. 312 para. 2). If A.I.D. is established, denial of paternity is possible even if the husband gave his consent—still with the reservation about possible damages—but because of the rules of medical secrecy a successful end to such an action is hypothetical. A suit for denial can be lodged only within six months after the birth.

Under these conditions, we think that French positive law is a sufficient guarantee to the people concerned in artificial insemination, and that no legislation is needed. The laws of affiliation ensure for the ensuing child a status similar to that of a legitimate child. The particular conditions of a child's conception should be no concern of the law, and this is why the confidentiality of such an intervention should be maintained in all cases.

This solution is not possible in all foreign legal systems. According to German law, affiliation can be contested after A.I.D. even if the husband has given his consent. A.I.D. is forbidden under Swiss law as being incompatible with the institution of marriage:[14] Swiss doctrine concludes that a child born as a result of A.I.D. can be disavowed (Art. 254 Swiss Civil Code). Only Portuguese law expressly considers artificial insemination: article 1799 of the Portuguese Civil Code provides that artificial fertilization is not a sufficient proof by itself in discussing affiliation.[20]

What would happen in France in a conflict between different legal systems? The number of children born from legitimate or illegitimate unions between individuals of different nationalities is increasing every year. French private international law has until now been based only on jurisprudence. The Decree of 3rd January 1972 was revolutionary in introducing into the Civil Code (Arts. 311.14–18) five articles relating to conflicts between legal systems in the matter of affiliation. These articles constitute a beginning in the codification of French private international law.[3]

Article 311.14 provides that affiliation is regulated by the mother's personal law on the day of the child's birth; if the mother is not known, by the child's personal law. Article 311.15 modifies the application of the mother's law: if the legitimate child and its father and mother, the natural child and its father or mother have their common or separate usual residence in France, the facts in proof of civil status will have all the consequences which would derive from French law, even if the other elements of affiliation could have depended on the foreign law. This ruling was motivated by considerations of family peace and its advantage is that it saves foreigners living in France from the consequences of the mother's foreign law.[21] Thus, the affiliation of a child born in France to foreign parents as a result of A.I.D. cannot be disputed in France provided the child has facts in proof of his civil status (*possession d'état*) and an identity deed.

Another category of conflicts concerns the division of medical responsibility into its elements in the law of torts and the law of contract. The torts are subject to the law of the country where these wrongs have taken place (*lex loci delicti*). From the point of view of liability in contract, the law of contract, which determines the obligations of the parties, must also fix the consequences of noncompliance with these obligations. If no choice is expressed by the parties, the law of the country where the contract is executed will be applied.[2] The determination of which legal system is the competent one is highly relevant. Certainly, the principles governing medical responsibility in French law differ from those in English and American law which, in some cases, bind the doctor to achieve a successful conclusion of the treatment. Exemption clauses (in the form of a signed permission for an operation) are allowed in the U.S.A. but forbidden in France.

Still more important differences apparently separate French law from foreign legislatures where maternal affiliation is to be established. In Germany, Switzerland, Austria and Poland, maternal affiliation stems directly from the fact of birth alone.[16] In France, legal elements (such as the name on the birth certificate or proof of civil status for illegitimate affiliation) are needed in addition to the fact of birth. What will be the consequences of biological techniques which throw doubt on maternal affiliation?

EMBRYO TRANSFER

The implantation of human embryos sets a number of psychological, moral and legal problems.[37] Since it is possible to fertilize a human egg *in vitro*, from what moment can the fertilized egg be considered as an individual? Can a future mother have her child borne by another? What would be the affiliation of a child genetically belonging to another woman than his mother?[32] As always, science precedes the law and such possibilities have not been considered by lawyers, who have been more preoccupied with parthenogenesis.[18] We now enter the realm of legal conjecture. We shall examine the possible legal problems resulting from embryo implantation in humans, a technique which has already been experimentally performed in animals.[12, 33] Our classification is based on the pathological conditions that prevent a woman from having children normally.

For example, Mrs Smith is sterile because of tubal obstruction—she can still ovulate—and she wants to have a child. After artificial induction of ovulation, her ova can be removed, fertilized *in vitro* with the husband's sperm and the fertilized egg implanted in her uterus. The doctor owes his patient a duty of care and cannot guarantee the desired fertilization. In principle, the operation entails no particular risk. At present, the risk to the foetus is neither known nor capable of evaluation; therefore we believe that the doctor is not professionally responsible if the child is born malformed. If he were to be held responsible, this would mean indirectly introducing a guarantee of a successful result, since any therapy carries risks which the interested parties should bear only when they are aware of that risk. The same conditions will apply for paternal affiliation as in A.I.H. Maternal affiliation, of course, is not in question.

Secondly, imagine Mrs A's sterility is of ovarian origin, and she wants a child. An anonymous female donor B is inseminated with Mr A's sperm. At implantation, the fertilized egg is taken out of B's womb and implanted into Mrs A's womb. This embryo transfer by donor is comparable to A.I.D. Anonymity will be strictly preserved. As in A.I.D., the doctor could be held responsible for choosing a highly unsuitable mother and for the transmission of a hereditary disease or infection. Maternal affiliation will be established by the birth certificate and paternal affiliation is in no doubt. Since maternity in France is established by confinement, Mrs A cannot contest the maternity of a child of whom she has been delivered. Conversely, if medical secrecy were violated, the egg donor B could not claim the child since she was not confined.

The third example covers more complex medical and aetiological situations: uterine malformation, malignant hypertension, congestive heart failure, chronic renal insufficiency, foeto-maternal isoimmunization, and rhesus incompatibility. The analysis of each is complicated by the necessity of comparing the risks to mother or foetus with those inherent in normal pregnancy. Chronic renal insufficiency can be treated by kidney transplant, and more than thirty women with kidney allografts have successfully given birth to a healthy child. However, in each case, the risks of rejection were considered to be increased by pregnancy. Similarly, a woman suffering from congestive heart failure can be treated surgically, but subsequent pregnancy could be fatal and the risk is difficult to evaluate accurately. The best solution in the cases listed above is removal of the embryo after normal fertilization by the husband, and implantation of the embryo in a mother, called a 'nurse'.[29] For example, Mrs Smith suffers from mitral stenosis; she is not sterile but pregnancy could aggravate her illness. Mrs Smith has an unmarried sister, Miss Jones, enjoying excellent health and willing to help. The implantation of Mrs Smith's ovum, fertilized by her husband, into Miss Jones would allow the Smiths to satisfy their wish for a child. Mrs Smith could share with her sister the waiting for this child borne by Miss Jones. This generous sister could become the child's godmother. Miss Jones has in no way contributed genetically to the child but only supplied the vital medium necessary to its development, just like a nurse who feeds a child entrusted to her.

Before such a thing could happen,[26] the motivations of this disinterested action should be examined, if necessary with the help of a psychiatrist. The precautions taken before a person agrees to be a kidney donor may, it seems, be applicable to the aforementioned situation, and we believe that embryo transfer represents an analogous psychological context, although the disability and its treatment remain very different. Moreover, it is not a matter of saving life, but of allowing a child to come into the world. The risks run by the nurse (womb-mother) are certainly no higher than those run by the donor of a kidney, the more so as this pregnancy would be induced only after a complete precautionary medical examination.

This situation results in a real legal imbroglio. The child should be declared at the Registry Office as born to Miss Jones since the link of maternal affiliation is established by confinement, and the nurse could keep the child. But what would happen if the Smiths refused to accept the child on account of which Miss Jones had been confined? Alternatively, the mother of the child could be declared unknown. The forsaken child would be taken into care, then adopted from birth by his own parents. This is illogical since genetically the child is the Smiths'. Finally, if it is decided to register the child under the Smiths' name, there would be a legal presumption of maternity although there was no confinement. This hypothetical situation has been considered: a woman who does not want to keep her child gives it to another who simulates confinement. This procedure allows avoidance of the rules of adoption.[13, 15, 22] This situation, which legally is quite abnormal, is biologically no more abnormal than the others and, further, it is as justifiable medically as artificial insemination is. Of course, the application of embryo transfer should be subservient to therapeutic considerations: any other motivation—coquetry, ambition or pursuit of a career where aesthetics are essential—should exclude such action. The publicity roused by these latter applications is enough to remind us that solutions which are therapeutically acceptable can become scandalous when there is no medical justification for them.

The last example considers both male and female sterility. Mrs Smith is sterile and cannot produce a viable ovum, although she could bear a child to term. Mr Smith is also sterile through incurable azoospermia. An anonymous donor couple supply the genetic material, having been selected by the doctor in the usual way. At the appropriate time, the donor embryo will be implanted in Mrs Smith's womb. Certainly, the resultant child does not genetically belong to the Smiths. As in A.I.D., the doctor is responsible for the choice of the donors and also if any harm, such as transmission of disease, occurs through negligence. Anonymity being the rule, Mrs Smith will be delivered of a legitimate child who benefits by the presumption *pater is est*. The donors have only given a fertilized egg and not a child, which is not prenatal surrender, although it is prenatal adoption by the beneficiary couple. Adoption being admitted, what objection can be made to this application of embryo implantation? What would happen if the identities of the embryo donors were divulged, or if they were to make the acquaintance of the beneficiary couple? Because of anonymity, these questions should not arise. Any further legal analysis seems to us intuitively absurd, although *in abstracto* the situation is not essentially different from the foregoing examples.

On the verge of its application to humans, embryo implantation should be discussed in the context of experimentation on humans. Any study of fertilized eggs is human experimentation and therefore subject to the limitations expressed by the Declaration of Helsinki. The only problem for the sperm donor is the religious interdiction of masturbation. Adequate precautions will be necessary during the removal of the donor's ova. Both her consent and knowledge of the medical purpose of the experiment are essential. The doctor should refuse to remove the ova if he has either to act clandestinely or neglect any possible psychological repercussions. In any human experiment, the individual's wishes must be respected, bearing in mind the psychological perturbation which any experiment touching on the origin of life could cause in imaginative and delicate minds.

So far as fertilization *in vitro* can be followed by embryonic development, it will be necessary one day to prescribe the limit beyond which the experimenter is no longer in the presence of a mass of cultivated cells but of a potential human being.

The interdictions formulated by lawyers and, more often, by theologians and moralists, about new therapies and especially the research work necessary to establish them, are only the expression of collective fear. Every time medicine has come up against taboos, there have been experimenters sufficiently bold and spirited to ignore them. Science advances through successive mutations, thanks to individuals who are intellectual revolutionaries. The scientist cannot accept the same morals as the lawyer, who often expresses popular convictions.

Conversely, throughout this paper, the justification of the recommended solution has always been based on a choice between a risk and therapeutic benefit for the individual. But my analysis tries to show a new category of risk, the moral risk, which appears as a chasm between the adopted solution and commonly admitted rules of behaviour. The juxtaposition of this attitude with the problems raised by experimentation on the human embryo shows up an essential limit at the level of motivation. Just as I consider that artificial insemination and embryo transfer are indefensible without the medical justification of the treatment of sterility, so I suggest that any experimentation on the fertilized egg with no specific medical purpose, that is simply to obtain a better knowledge of the biology and pathology of the human embryo, should be condemned. Any experimental procedure trying to find the solution of problems which could be solved by experiments on animals seems unjustifiable to us. However, I am aware of the possible usefulness of an experimental approach to the human embryo and realize the difficulties raised if an immediate therapeutic purpose is assigned to fundamental research which, often unforeseeably, can be most useful to medicine. This stresses the moral level which we are entitled to demand of the scientist perhaps more than of the therapist himself.

ACKNOWLEDGEMENTS

I thank Dr M. Cognat (Lyon) who made his technical experience of the field available, and Mr J. Massip, Magistrat au Ministère de la Justice (Direction des Affaires Civiles et du Sceau), and Mr G. Morin (Rédacteur en Chef au Répertoire du Notariat) who kindly reviewed the manuscript. I am also grateful to Dr J. P. Revillard for stimulating discussions and invaluable suggestions.

References

[1] AUBREY, L. & RAU, C. (1962) Droit Civil Français, Vol. VIII, Esmein & Ponsard, Paris
[2] BATIFFOL, H. (1971) Droit International Privé, 5th edn., Libraire Générale de Droit et de Jurisprudence, Paris
[3] BATIFFOL, H. & LAGARDE, P. (1972) L'improvisation de nouvelles règles de conflits de lois en matière de filiation. Revue Critique de Droit International Privé, 1–26
[4] BRETON, A. (1956) note sous Lyon 28 Mai 1956 D. 1956J.646
[5] Cahiers Laënnec (1948) L'insémination artificielle, Lethielleux, Paris
[6] COHEN, J. (1972) Les Stérilités Masculines en Pratique Gynécologique, Masson, Paris
[7] DASTE, M. (1948) Les conséquences juridiques en droit civil français de l'insémination artificielle. Annales de Médecine Légale, 225–261
[8] DECOCQ, A. (1960) Essai d'une Théorie Générale des Droits sur la Personne, Librairie Générale de Droit et de Jurisprudence, Paris
[9] DIERKENS, R. (1966) Les Droits sur le Corps et le Cadavre de l'Homme, Collection de Médecine Légale, Paris
[10] DOLL, P. J. (1970) La Discipline des Greffes, des Transplantations et des Autres Actes de Disposition Concernant le Corps Humain, Masson, Paris
[11] DÖLLE, H. (1965) Familienrecht, Vol. II, p. 46, Müller, Karlsruhe
[12] EDWARDS, R. G., BAVISTER, B. D. & STEPTOE, P. C. (1969) Early stages of fertilization in vitro of human oocytes matured in vitro. Nature (London) 221, 632–635
[13] GEBLER, M. J. (1970) Le Droit Français de la Filiation et la Vérité, Librairie Générale de Droit et de Jurisprudence, Paris
[14] GROSSEN, J. M. (1960) La Protection de la Personnalité en Droit Privé (rapport présenté à la Société Suisse des Juristes), No. 62, pp. 51a–52a, Helbing & Lichtenhahn, Basel
[15] HOLLEAUX, G. (1942) note sous Aix 20 Novembre 1940 DC 1942–85

[16] HOLLEAUX, G. (1966) *De la Filiation en Droit Allemand, Suisse et Français: essais de droit comparé*, Cujas, Paris

[17] Instruction générale relative à l'Etat Civil (1970), *Journal Officiel*

[18] KORNPROBST, L. (1957) *Responsabilité du Médecin devant la Loi et la Jurisprudence Françaises*, Flammarion, Paris

[19] LEBECH, P. E. (1972) *Banques de Spermes Humains: fécondité et stérilité du mâle*, Colloque de la Société Nationale pour l'Étude de la Stérilité et de la Fécondité, 2nd edn., Masson, Paris

[20] LISBONNE, J. (1967) *Jurisclasseur de Droit Comparé. V Portugal*, editions Techniques, Paris

[21] MASSIP, J., MORIN, G. & AUBERT, J. L. (1972) *La Réforme de la Filiation* (commentaire de la loi du 3 Janvier 1972, préface de J. Carbonnier), Répertoire du Notariat Defrénois, Paris

[22] MAZEAUD, H. L. J. (1959) *Leçons de Droit Civil*, Vol. I, p. 862, Montchrestien, Paris

[23] MERGER, R. (1957) L'insémination artificielle. *La Semaine Juridique* 1, 1389

[24] MORIN, M. (1967) *La Réforme de l'Adoption* (loi du 11 Juillet 1966), Répertoire du Notariat Defrénois, Paris

[25] NERSON, R. (1970) L'influence de la biologie et de la médecine moderne sur le droit civil, *Revue Trimestrielle de Droit Civil*, 661–683

[26] PARKES, SIR A. (1972) quoted in *Nature (London)* 238, 241

[27] PISAPIA, G. D. (1962) Les problèmes de droit pénal posés par l'insémination artificielle. *Revue de Science Criminelle et de Droit Penal Comparé*, 47–64

[28] PONSARD, A. (1962) *Les Techniques Biologiques et le Droit de la Famille* (Conférence donnée au Centre Européen Universitaire de Nancy en Mars 1962), unpublished

[29] RADOVIC, P. (1971) Possibility of treatment of sterility in woman by transplantation of the fertilized oocyte (VIIth World Congress on Fertility and Sterility, Tokyo), Abstract 153, International Congress Series No. 234, Excerpta Medica, Amsterdam

[30] REVILLARD, M. & REVILLARD, J. P. (1966) Les aspects juridiques des transplantations d'organes chez l'homme. *Revue Lyonnaise de Médecine* 13, 21–23

[31] REVILLARD, M. & REVILLARD, J. P. (1972) Problèmes de responsabilité juridique liés à l'utilisation de matériel de réanimation médicale. *Agressologie* 13, 21–31

[32] RORVIK, D. (1971) *Brave New Baby*, Doubleday, New York and (1972) Albin Michel, Paris

[33] STEPTOE, P. C., EDWARDS, R. G. & PURDY, J. M. (1971) Human blastocysts grown in culture. *Nature (London)* 229, 132–133

[34] SAVATIER, R. (1948) *Le Droit Civil de la Famille et les Conquêtes de la Biologie*, Ch. 33, Dalloz, Paris

[35] SAVATIER, R., AUBY, J. M. & PEQUIGNOT, H. (1956) *Traité de Droit Médical* §253, 254–277

[36] THELIN, M. T. (1947) L'insémination artificielle. *Annales de Médecine Légale*, 209–216

[37] THIBAULT, C. (1971) La fécondation *in vitro*. *Concours Médical* 93, 6695–6702

[38] Travaux de la Commission de Réforme du Code Civil (1950–1951) *Insémination Artificielle*, pp. 164–168, Sirey, Paris

Discussion: legal aspects

Kilbrandon: I shall be immediately disclosed as an old-fashioned 'Benthamite utilitarian', because I still hold to the view that the law should not forbid what it is not necessary to forbid and, so far as possible, it ought to authorize what people feel they want to do. We have spoken much about both the machinery of the law and more serious things. In general (this is why I am going to try and take a utilitarian view) we must try to consider with whom we are dealing. The essential unreality of the Feversham Report was that it did not deal with a problem which is relevant to most people.

One conclusion which has come out of this symposium so far is that the acceptance of A.I.D. and the facilitation of it in one sense emphasize the importance of the family concept. In relation to the A.I.D. child, the father becomes the joint head of the family, whether or not he is the actual father of the child. The family as an entity is concentrated on, rather than the actual paternity or maternity; physical paternity is seen to take second place to some kind of a community relation. An example is when a married couple take over the child of a dead brother and his wife. Such children become part of the family, and then there is a community relationship; in that family it does not matter who is the mother and who is the father—that becomes irrelevant. As Professor Williams emphasized, the *pater familias* is much more important than the actual genetic father.

Miss Stone said that by the law of Scotland, A.I.D. without the consent of the wife is not adultery (p. 69), and that is certainly the present position.[1] There is some authority in an English case in the House of Lords[2] from which it may be inferred that it is: but it is a matter of no importance now. I agree that such action could undoubtedly be treated by the courts as conduct rendering it impossible for the marriage to continue, and thus to have broken down irretrievably. Then Miss Stone raised the interesting question of what action a mother might be able to take against a doctor after A.I.D. The mother is in one of two relationships with the doctor: a relationship of contract and a relationship arising out of the doctor's duty to take reasonable care in giving her treatment for which she has asked. If the doctor were to contract to produce the semen of, say, a six-foot-tall blond and the mother did not get that, I do not know whether she would have an action for breach of contract. If she received semen from, say, somebody with a congenital disease and no proper precautions had been taken, I have no doubt she would have an action of damages in negligence. I assembled a number of authorities on the child's relationship with the doctor for the conference in October 1971 that I mentioned earlier (p. 1). The first case mentioned there was of a pregnant married woman who was given a blood transfusion and, by the carelessness of the hospital, was given blood infected with syphilis. She gave birth to a syphilitic girl. This child was held to have an action of damages against the hospital, in negligence; that is obvious. But in other cases children brought actions of damages against their parents for infecting them with venereal disease. An Italian court allowed an action of damages in these circumstances, and so did a lower German court, but the *Bundesgericht* would not allow it, because they said that this damage arose from the act of conception which was what brought the plaintiff into the world. Now, that may be right or not; it has been followed in the American courts. But we are in a different situation with A.I.D., because the child would be able to say 'I was not born of sexual intercourse at all. I was born from the act of a doctor, who took semen out of the wrong bottle, and he is liable to me for the neglect of a duty of care which he owed to me'. There might be a distinction here from the cases referred to (I think there probably is); we cannot assume that the child would not have a right of action against the doctor and perhaps the hospital services responsible. That is truly a fundamental civil rights aspect of the matter.

We must not make too much of the registration of the birth. We cannot say that a child born of A.I.D. is legitimate within the meaning of the word now. We must simply change the meaning of the word 'legitimate', if we want to turn this child into a legitimate child—and a great deal is to be said for changing the meaning. After all, the child is legitimate in that it was borne by the wife, in fulfilment of the wishes of the husband, and, in that sense, to call it illegitimate is a misuse of language. When it comes to registration, no question of principle is involved. It is sometimes overlooked that maternity is a question of fact, but paternity is only an inference. No one can prove paternity, whereas maternity can be proved by the evidence of witnesses. So that the decision about what goes into the register in the 'father' column is in that sense always a matter of opinion. There seems to be no case for registering a child as 'father unknown', although that depends on what our recommendations are going to be in other fields. Are we going to recommend that the donor is to be known? Is there to be a register of donors as there is a register of adoptions? If not, and especially if there are to be mixed semen banks, then the father *is* unknown, but otherwise the father might not be unknown. I suggest that the heading of one of the columns of the register be changed so that children are registered in the name of 'father or accepting husband'. It would not matter then whether the conception was normal or as a result of A.I.D.

Fortunately, embryo transfer from the woman and back to her is apparently a 'non-problem'. It occurred to me that it is analogous to a Caesarean birth: simply an artificial means of organizing an ordinary birth, thus raising no extraordinary social or legal aspects.

Madame Revillard, I did not know that in France a couple cannot adopt a child if they have natural children of their own.

Revillard: The essential condition for adoption in French law is the absence of any legitimate descendant, except in special circumstances where authorization has been accorded by the President of the Republic (art. 345–1). Conversely, having an illegitimate acknowledged child did not formerly prevent the parents from adopting another child unless the first had been legitimated. Now that the law of affiliation has been reformed to give the illegitimate acknowledged child the same rights as a legitimate child, the question of whether a person who has an illegitimate acknowledged child can adopt a child would seem to need reconsideration.

Kilbrandon: That is not the law in this country. There is something to be said for having a rule that a woman cannot have children by A.I.D. if she already has natural children, although I can see that might raise complications.

I am delighted that the French have been so sensible as to say that a birth to the woman after she and her husband have been separated for more than 300 days is illegitimate (p. 83). We have no such rule yet. In one unfortunate case a child born 340 days after separation was accepted as legitimate, to the laughter of the whole medical profession!

R. G. Edwards: The role of the third party in achieving a conception seems to be central to the topic of this symposium. Few rules cover this unless the child is born with or develops an anomaly. For example, the hormone treatment sometimes needed to induce a woman to ovulate is just as much an interference as is A.I.D. or A.I.H. Without such interference, there is no child. Embryo transfer raises similar issues. Is there any law or are there any cases which would clarify the legal position of the third party?

Kilbrandon: The procedures you described and those we have been discussing are simply to be classified as legitimate surgical interferences. Their nature or purpose does not matter provided that it is legitimate, and nobody has ever suggested that these interferences are not legitimate. The ordinary law applies. It seems to be the same as if a surgeon were taking out the woman's appendix.

R. G. Edwards: If a child born as a result of A.I.H. is deformed, what is the situation then? Of course, without an act, there would be no conception. But, for example, in the case of the child born with syphilis (p. 92), what was the relation between the father who was infected, the doctor who did the insemination and the child? Could the child claim damages from the doctor?

Kilbrandon: Yes, *if* the doctor knew or ought to have known that he was inseminating the woman from a syphilitic husband.

Stone: If he did not know, he was negligent.

Stallworthy: Surely there are two separate points? If the child is born a congenital syphilitic, it does not necessarily follow that it was infected at the time of its conception. It could be very difficult to prove in retrospect that an A.I.D. father did or did not have syphilis before insemination. Any doctor responsible for a woman's antenatal care who finds later that she produced a congenitally syphilitic child would have no medico-legal defence. He should discover her infection during pregnancy and give the treatment necessary to safeguard both the mother and the foetus. The child is born with a preventable disease but it would be necessary to prove that infection took place at conception. It could happen later in pregnancy.

J. H. Edwards: These procedures are slightly different from taking an appendix out, because if anything goes wrong in that operation it is likely that expert witnesses will be called to explain the hazards of taking an appendix out (and of not taking it out). The doctor could be held to have not reasonably acted otherwise. One can treat an embryo very severely, for instance by giving vast doses of hormones to diagnose pregnancy, which is one particularly curious technique which appears to be legal, or by mechanical operations, such as removing an embryo and storing it *in vitro* for three weeks, which in the opinion of some experts is likely to cause trouble. How would that stand in the face of expert testimony in law?

Kilbrandon: Unfortunately there would be a row of experts on each side. The judge must decide.

J. H. Edwards: With established surgical procedures, experts would agree that the surgeon made an error but that the act was in good faith, whereas, if something went wrong during embryo transfer, one might be able to produce a majority of experts who could say that, in their opinion, this was the sort of tragedy which was predictable.

Kilbrandon: I am only saying that the *law* is the same in both cases. The law is that if the doctor does something which is not in accordance with common professional procedures and damage is caused, then that is negligence. That is easy to prove in some cases and difficult in others.

J. H. Edwards: But if it is a completely new treatment, as in thalidomide tragedies, you cannot get evidence without catastrophic consequences. In law, do you have to produce practical evidence for expert prognostications?

Kilbrandon: In the first case, expert opinion would be called upon to determine the question 'would a careful doctor have done this?' That is what it amounts to.

Steptoe: What is the legal position of the doctor who initiates a pregnancy by embryo transfer in good faith, believing that he is going to produce a normal pregnancy, and then finds that an abnormal child is born?

Kilbrandon: It would depend whether there was any means by which he could have found this out.

Steptoe: But, as Professor Edwards just said, these are brand new procedures with no previous experience to benefit from.

Kilbrandon: Was the child abnormal in consequence of the procedure?

Steptoe: That would be unknown, because there is an incidence of abnormality anyway.

Kilbrandon: Anybody challenging the doctor would have to make out their case. The onus of proof would be on them. Unless it could be shown that the doctor had been negligent there would be no action against him.

Bevis: The mass media are hysterically interested in embryo transfer in particular. This seems to be the major ethical problem at the moment. Suppose that the position Dr Steptoe outlined arose, the mass media found out, and the accusing finger of the world was pointed at the child, how would the doctor stand there?

Kilbrandon: How could anybody point a finger at the child after an embryo transplant? It is a legitimate child which has been produced by a legitimate surgical interference.

Stallworthy: Could the position perhaps be clarified by the doctors themselves making it perfectly clear to people consenting to an experiment that they are doing this knowingly and accepting the implications which may be inherent in their action? One of the unfortunate things about the brilliant work of Edwards and Steptoe has been the adverse publicity in the mass media. This is evident when you see an unhappy woman speaking on television, obviously believing that she will soon undergo a simple procedure which will provide her with the baby she desires. Because of their deep emotional involvement these are the people who, if something goes wrong, are likely to raise medico-legal problems. However, I am sure Drs Edwards and Steptoe have received many letters, such as those that some of us who are also interested in the study of fertility receive, saying, for example, 'I am a doctor and I know of this fertility research. Has it got to the stage when it could be of any use to me because above everything else in life I want a baby and I am prepared to accept the risks?' Some people make statements like this in their original letters asking for help. These letters constitute a safeguard against subsequent legal proceedings.

Kilbrandon: I do not know how far a release by the parents would bind the child.

Steptoe: We do take all these precautions of course, and we believe also that the modern methods of monitoring pregnancy will exclude any serious abnormality.

J. H. Edwards: When we discussed the biological situation, the distinction was drawn between genetic and cultural family relationships. There was anxiety (which there are good grounds for regarding as minimal) that incest would take place unknowingly without genetic registers. Is incest a cultural or a genetic relation as the law stands now?

Kilbrandon: An incestuous act of intercourse is a crime. It is provided by the Adoption Act, 1958, s. 13(3), that an adoptive parent is, for purposes of marriage, deemed to be within the prohibited degree of consanguinity in relation to an adopted child. It is an open question whether intercourse between, say, an adoptive father and his adopted daughter is incest.

Stone: It is desirable, and usual in English law, to make a distinction and talk about incest only in terms of the criminal law. The prohibited degrees of marriage in the civil law simply mean that people within those degrees cannot validly marry each other but they have not necessarily committed any criminal offence if they have sexual intercourse. The Sexual Offences Act, 1956, s.10(1), declares it a criminal offence for a man to have sexual intercourse with a woman whom he knows to be his grand-daughter, daughter, sister or mother. Sister includes half-sister, and illegitimate relationships apply as well as legitimate. In section 11 of that Act, corresponding offences are declared for a woman having sexual intercourse with her grandfather, father, brother or son. That is the criminal offence of incest. It is interesting that there is a prohibition on an adopter marrying the child whom he has adopted. This illustrates that prohibition of marriage exists for social as well as for genetic reasons. The marriage prohibition goes no further than adopter and adopted. The Stockdale Committee on adoption and long-term fostering considered whether there should be a prohibition of marriage between an adopted child and a natural child of his adopter, and in its Report[3] the Committee discusses the arguments and concludes that it is not necessary for the prohibition to be extended. For example, a woman, Jane, adopts a boy, John. Jane can never validly marry John. But if Jane had a daughter, Nancy, John can validly marry Nancy. The Stockdale Committee considered whether such a marriage should be prohibited, and decided that it should not. Confusion sometimes arises because the Americans tend to talk about incest in civil law as well; we do not.

Kilbrandon: Incest was not even a crime in England until 1908.

Stone: It was a crime in the church courts, which had a much wider definition of incest.

Andrejew: The legal system in Poland is somewhat different, and obviously I will not be able to go into the details of how it differs. We consider incest as a crime; it covers sexual intercourse not only between relatives but also between the adopter and the adopted. Our system differs so much that, for instance, we have no legal notion of legitimate and illegitimate children. We have no legal notion of adultery. When a child is born within a marriage, the husband is presumed to be the father and the child is registered as the child of the couple. The husband may claim not to be the father within a period of six months from the moment he knows of the child's birth. If he does not do that, he remains the father of the child in the view of the law. In recent years, we had several interesting decisions by the Supreme Court that, in my opinion, look forward to the future. On several occasions, the Supreme Court found that the mere fact of the biological impossibility of the child being the child of the husband is not sufficient to deny paternity. What is important is the well-being and social situation of the child, not the biological aspect. In one case, a couple took a child from a maternity hospital and registered it as their own. The woman was not the mother of the child, nor was the man the father. After many years the man stopped loving the woman and wanted to get out of the affair. He claimed before the court that the woman was not the mother of the child, but the court refused to accept this: it said that the mere biological impossibility was not a sufficient ground.

Looking to the future, I see the problem of granting a woman the possibility of acting according to her biological vocation. If she cannot have a child from her husband, arrangements should be made for her to be inseminated, provided the husband agrees, and the child should be considered as the child of the couple. Otherwise she might be pushed to commit adultery or to be inseminated under improper conditions that could do her harm. I feel that this should be the primary aspect rather than the comparatively petty difficulties that arise. The best way of procreation is natural intercourse; everybody realizes that! Certainly there are many difficulties, but we have to approach the social problem as it is and find a reasonable solution.

Piattelli-Palmarini: Two aspects in Catholic practice and in church law are worth mention. First, the only exception to the law against abortion is in the case of rape (see p. 20), when the woman has the right to remove the product of this undesired fertilization by mild methods.

The second point comes not from canonical law but from the ethical views of Catholic doctors. The prevailing ethics once were such that whenever a couple could not have children, the doctor was advised preferably not to inform them about which partner was sterile or infertile, for since the marriage was indissoluble and no other way of having children was then known, no purpose was served. More recently, as treatment for infertility has become more successful, the attitudes of the Catholic doctor have changed so that although the identity of the infertile partner may still not be revealed, the doctor will at least investigate the couple. If the infertility could be successfully treated, the doctor would feel that he had the right to tell both partners. However, with incurable infertility, I believe the Catholic doctor prefers not to tell the couple which of them is responsible.

McLaren: I understood Miss Stone to say that with the law as it is at present it is not possible to renounce parental rights and duties. Surely the original parents of an adopted child renounce their rights and duties?

Stone: Because the parents cannot effectively renounce their rights and duties there can be no adoption until the court has actually made the adoption order. By the Adoption Act, 1958, s.13(1), 'Upon an adoption order being made, all rights, duties, obligations and liabilities of the parents or guardians of the infant ... shall be extinguished, and all such rights, duties, obligations and liabilities shall vest in and be exercisable by and enforceable against the adopter as if the infant were a child born to the adopter in lawful wedlock ...'. That is why up to the very moment that the adoption order is made the parents may resile from the consent previously given. After the order is made, it vests parental rights in the adopter. Also, of course, the question might arise whether the parents are unreasonably withholding or withdrawing their consent, or whether for any other reason their consent may be dispensed with.

McLaren: I understand that in this country the rights of the adopted child are in no way different from those of an ordinary child with respect to the inheritance of property. However, may an A.I.D. child technically have a claim on the sperm donor's estate if the donor dies intestate or bequeaths money to his children?

Stone: First, you cannot say there is no difference; for the adopted child's rights to succession I refer you to the Adoption Act, 1958, s.15 and 16. The net effect—and this was the intention—is probably that he is in the same position as the ordinary child. But of course, since 1970, by the Family Law Reform Act, 1969, s.14, so also is the illegitimate child on intestacy; he is 'entitled to take any interest ... to which he ... would have been entitled if he had been born legitimate' if either of his parents dies leaving property and no will. Also the word child now does not mean legitimate child only as it did until 1970. As regards the sperm donor, the child would have to prove that he was the child of this particular person. He has no presumptions to help him; this is the difficulty of any illegitimate child. He must prove that X was his father, which obviously is going to be a difficult matter as regards the sperm donor. But in theory, if the child could prove this to the satisfaction of the court, he would have a right to succession.

Kilbrandon: This is going to cause consternation in Dr Mason's clinic, because all her donors are going to be liable to support all their children.

Stone: Dr McLaren was asking about actual succession to the property of a parent who has died, which is rather different from maintenance.

Kilbrandon: Intestate donors will be liable to having their estates split up among all the people they fathered.

Mason: There should be no way in which the identity of the donor can be discovered.

Dunstan: Couldn't the court subpoena the doctor to produce the records?

Kilbrandon: If you are going to keep a record of donors for genetic purposes, this could probably arise.

Stallworthy: Recently a leading international research worker in this country had a subpoena served on him to produce a confidential record of his research, because lawyers in the U.S. were able to get the necessary legal permission to do this. The case will be fought if necessary up to the highest level, especially as the protection societies concerned have accepted responsibility for defending him.

Fried: I think Miss Stone's suggestion that A.I.D. children be treated as adopted children is really very bad advice. By far the simpler solution would be the one which she described as the California solution, where, if the husband has consented, that child is for all purposes considered as the child of both parties to the marriage.

I have been told I should have an almost Germanic respect for the accuracy of the register of births. The inaccuracy of the register does not seem to pose a great problem, unless it is for scientific research and then it is possible that medical records could be kept which would allow such accuracy to be maintained, if that is important. If the law is about to be reformed in England, then by far the best thing would be for the matter to be simplified, because under Miss Stone's solution the husband could decide, eight or nine months later, that he will not adopt this child, which would be somewhat awkward.

McLaren: The ambiguous position of the A.I.D. child with respect to the inheritance of property from the sperm donor and from the 'stepfather' seems a major anomaly in the law at present. I would like to see the A.I.D. child at least on a par with the adopted child from this point of view. Could Miss Stone's suggestion about prenatal adoption be incorporated in the husband's consent to A.I.D.? Could his consent be considered as a form of *de jure* adoption, rather than a quite separate legal procedure having to be gone through later?

Stone: The law is clear at the moment: no one can apply to adopt a child until the child is four and a half months old. Therefore I was suggesting that it would be an improvement if an application to adopt could be made at the time of the artificial insemination, and that an adoption order could be made contingent on the child being born alive. It seems to me that this would improve the position of the child. I was surprised that Professor Fried thought it was a horrible suggestion and that this was a much worse situation for the child. I don't understand that. What I was suggesting was that as soon as this child lets out his first scream, he will do so as an adopted child and not a child in respect of whom people have now to start going through legal procedures.

Fried: Clearly what you suggest would be an improvement, since of the present legal situation one might say yet again 'the law is a ass'. But it is so evidently a most tortuous half-measure, when the reasonable solution is the one Lord Kilbrandon suggested, which is just to say that if the husband has consented, then it is as if he had had intercourse with his wife and the child is the child of the marriage.

Kilbrandon: I must counter the impression that the A.I.D. child is going to be in the fortunate testamentary position of having two fathers, because I am sure this is not the case.

Dunstan: I am disappointed that I seem to be the only non-conservative here in that my plea for the abolition of the concept of illegitimacy has not been pursued.

Kilbrandon: Although I think the concept of illegitimacy is outside our terms of reference, I am fully prepared to defend your position, Canon Dunstan.

Stone: I agree; I am heartily in favour of doing away with the whole concept of an illegitimate child. In my view there are no illegitimate children, but only illegitimate parents. This is really the concept which we should consider. The parents cause the birth of this child out of wedlock and therefore it is the parents' so-called rights, if any, which should be diminished.

Dunstan: This is a blatant transferance of epithet.

Fielding: How far is it possible to determine the obligations of a doctor in the procedure of A.I.D.? And if there is agreement on certain important issues, is there need to seek some further sanctions outside the profession? New provisions in the criminal code have been suggested but were not thought to be helpful, perhaps being even harmful. Could any statutory provisions support the ethics of the profession if there were sufficient agreement and public acceptance?

Not long ago I found myself on a panel organized by some social workers in a

Canadian city. The purpose was to explore some of the problems presented to social workers by the practice of A.I.D. I based my opening remarks on the assumption, among others, that semen would be accepted only from a selected donor who had been carefully assessed at least with respect to the objective data of his medical and genetic history. A medical panelist seemed to feel that this assumption was a little naive on my part. His own practice, he said, was to ask one of his interns, who would bring the semen the next day and in exchange receive $25. At that time and place this appeared to be a perfectly acceptable practice. How much agreement is there about the proper medical procedure in selecting donors? If that question is important and if there is reasonable agreement, my next question is whether any statutory provision might help to support it.

Another panelist on the above occasion noted that sometimes he suspected that his would-be patients sought A.I.D. as an alibi for adultery. While he would not, of course, cooperate in the deceit if he could detect it, he apparently questioned paternity in some cases. Another panelist, in view of this, wondered whether 'adultery' with the consent of the husband and approval of the sub-culture might not be a simpler solution in some marriages than A.I.D. Here too there would seem to be many difficulties about establishing an accurate biological record of the facts.

In such situations we are faced with uncertainties about paternity or possibly serious hesitation about recording it. However, this uncertainty and these difficulties only reflect on a small scale (perhaps an insignificant scale) the same problems in society as a whole. Where no A.I.D. is involved, how sure are we of paternity in how large a segment of the population? The desire for privacy is normal; in addition deceit is easy. Much of the secrecy would be unveiled by blood tests, but not all. How can accurate biological records be kept in these circumstances? For example we have heard from Mr Philipp (p. 63) of one instance when about 30% of a group of babies could not possibly have been the children of their apparent fathers.

Kilbrandon: I am glad you raised the first point, because the procedure of A.I.D. sounds to me so simple that I should have thought it could be carried out by any competent midwife. I was assuming that A.I.D. would be carefully supervised in hospital.

Mason: I believe that there ought to be some legislation requiring that only a doctor should perform A.I.D.

Kilbrandon: Then we are running into the criminal law, aren't we?

Feilding: Is it conceivable that, either by the prevailing medical ethics or by statutory regulation, it might be considered malpractice to artificially inseminate anybody without first having conducted the proper tests as to the suitability of the donor's semen?

Kilbrandon: This would be better left to professional ethics rather than to the criminal law, which is a terrible blunderbuss. The trouble is that the practitioners need not be responsible for professional ethics, nor be qualified doctors.

Mason: It could be done perfectly legally by a nurse.

Himmelweit: We began by assuming that A.I.D. was only used in cases where there was proven sterility on the part of the man and careful investigation of suitability of semen used in A.I.D. Professor Feilding has shown that these two conditions do not always obtain. This might be even more applicable in the future, partly because the technique is so easy and partly because the reasons which make women want A.I.D., for example impatience for a child, may lead to requests for A.I.D. without extensive tests on the husband. This does suggest a need to register the practitioners, not because of the medical problems but because of problems of 'non-consent', that is, the husband might not have been consulted or indeed informed but might believe the child to be his own. Moreover another problem of non-consent is that the necessary careful selection of the donor might not be made.

Kilbrandon: I do not see that that conclusion follows.

Williams: We have come full circle. The next step is to allow natural insemination by a donor.

Steptoe: That would be adultery. Many patients do not regard A.I.D. as adultery.

Williams: But with the change in attitude which Professor Himmelweit was sketching, this might become acceptable.

Kilbrandon: I don't think the attitude has changed: the consent of the husband has underlain the whole discussion.

Himmelweit: All I am saying is that in the light of Professor Feilding's examples and the ease of the technique, one can imagine a variety of situations in which the woman could act without the consent of the husband. The question is whether it makes sense to tie the act of artificial insemination to the consent of the husband. This may not be possible.

Mason: But the lawyers have told us (pp. 69, 70, 91) that if the wife underwent A.I.D. without the consent of the husband, the husband might have grounds for divorce.

Himmelweit: It is also true that doctors in England will only perform A.I.D. with the husband's consent, and only when sterility is established.

Kilbrandon: There are worse forms of sexual activity than A.I.D. without the husband's consent, so why do we get so excited about it? If one indulges in these forms of sexual activity one might find oneself in the Divorce Court, but I do not see any reason why the couple or the doctor should find themselves in the Criminal Court for practising A.I.D. As Dr Steptoe said, most people will not go in for it, but those who do are responsible people.

Asked 'What do you think of sex?', Marilyn Monroe replied 'I think sex is here to stay!' I think that A.I.D. is here to stay. This symposium has been about what the law should do about it. The conclusion seems to be that the law has got to consider A.I.D. not in a prohibitory way and perhaps only in a regulatory way so far as is required to make the technique acceptable to society.

References

1   *Maclennan* v. *Maclennan* [1958] *S.C.* 105
2   *Russell* v. *Russell* [1924] *A.C.* 687 at p.721
3   Report of the Stockdale Committee (1972), Cmnd. 5107, para. 329–332, H.M. Stationery
        Office, London

Index of contributors

Entries in **bold** type indicate papers; other entries are contributions to discussions

Indexes compiled by William Hill.

Subject index